Illustrated Epidemiology

Jalal Poorolajal

Illustrated Epidemiology

A Visual Guide

Springer

Jalal Poorolajal
Department of Epidemiology, School of Public Health
Hamadan University of Medical Sciences
Hamadan, Iran

ISBN 978-981-96-9565-2 ISBN 978-981-96-9566-9 (eBook)
https://doi.org/10.1007/978-981-96-9566-9

This Springer imprint is published by the registered company Springer Nature Singapore Pte Ltd.
The registered company address is: 152 Beach Road, #21-01/04 Gateway East, Singapore 189721, Singapore

To Nahid

Preface

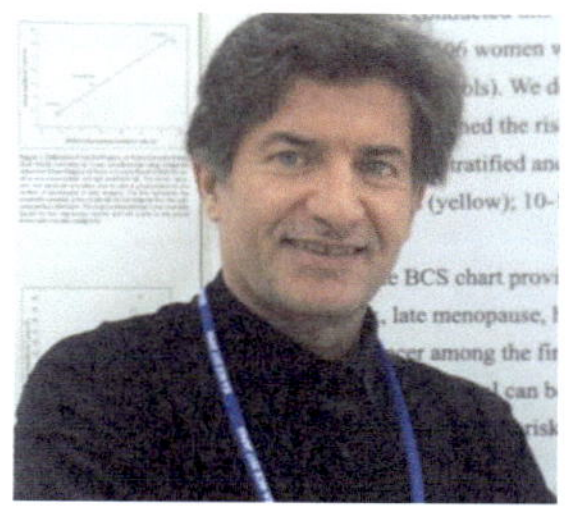

Epidemiology plays a pivotal role in promoting and protecting public health by elucidating the reasons behind illnesses, the mechanisms of disease transmission, and, most importantly, the strategies for prevention. Through the identification and management of factors contributing to disease outbreaks and their spread, epidemiology significantly enhances the quality and longevity of human life. Although it may appear to be a highly specialized field, the principles of epidemiology are accessible to anyone with an interest in health. The book *Illustrated Epidemiology: A Visual Guide* aims to simplify the learning process by presenting core epidemiological principles in a clear and concise manner, supported by visuals such as diagrams and illustrations.

My fascination with the power of visual aids in education began during my medical school years. The detailed and visually striking depictions by A.D.A.M. (Animated Dissection of Anatomy for Medicine) profoundly influenced my understanding of disease concepts and clinical manifestations, fostering a lifelong interest in visual communication. During my PhD studies in epidemiology, I observed a notable gap in the way complex epidemiological concepts were conveyed; they were often presented primarily in textual form, with insufficient reliance on visual aids. This observation inspired me to reimagine these intricate ideas as engaging, easy-to-understand visuals. Despite the availability of numerous textbooks on epidemiology, this visual approach has remained largely underutilized. With years of experience as an educator, I am now positioned to address this unmet need.

Visuals are uniquely effective as educational tools because they can simplify complex concepts and make them more comprehensible and memorable than text alone. They leave a lasting impression, enhancing both understanding and retention. For this reason, *Illustrated Epidemiology: A Visual Guide* leverages visuals to elucidate key epidemiological principles.

This book focuses on the fundamental concepts of epidemiology, avoiding overly technical jargon to ensure that readers can grasp the material with ease. Once the foundational concepts are understood, readers are encouraged to delve deeper into advanced topics through more specialized texts.

Hamadan, Iran
January 2025

Jalal Poorolajal

Acknowledgments

I would like to acknowledge the Department of Epidemiology, School of Public Health; the Modeling of Noncommunicable Diseases Research Center; and the Research Center for Health Sciences at Hamadan University of Medical Sciences for providing a supportive academic environment during the preparation of this book. The content of this book was developed independently and without any financial support.

Contents

Basic Concepts of Epidemiology

1

Contents

1.1 Prevention

Description

Prevention in epidemiology involves strategies designed to reduce the occurrence of diseases, injuries, or disabilities within a population. It focuses on proactively identifying and addressing risk factors to protect public health. There are primarily four levels of prevention, as illustrated in Fig. 1.1. While these levels are distinct, there is often considerable overlap, depending on the specific disease or condition [1–4].

Primordial Prevention

Primordial prevention is the earliest stage of disease prevention. It focuses on preventing the *emergence* of *risk factors* themselves, rather than targeting specific diseases. It involves creating a healthy environment and social conditions that minimize the occurrence of risk factors for disease.

One notable example of primordial prevention is the STRIP study, which was initiated in Finland in 1990. This study focused on counseling children from infancy to adolescence regarding healthy dietary habits. It emphasized the importance of consuming healthful fats; increasing the intake of fruits, vegetables, and whole grains; and reducing sodium consumption. By promoting healthy lifestyle choices during childhood, the STRIP study demonstrated a significant reduction in the prevalence of risk factors within the population. This ultimately contributed to a decrease in the incidence of cardiovascular diseases and an overall enhancement of public health [5].

In the context of hypertension, primordial prevention aims to implement early interventions to prevent the development of risk factors for high blood pressure, particularly during childhood and the prenatal period. Key strategies include promoting healthy eating habits,

J. Poorolajal, *Illustrated Epidemiology*, https://doi.org/10.1007/978-981-96-9566-9_1

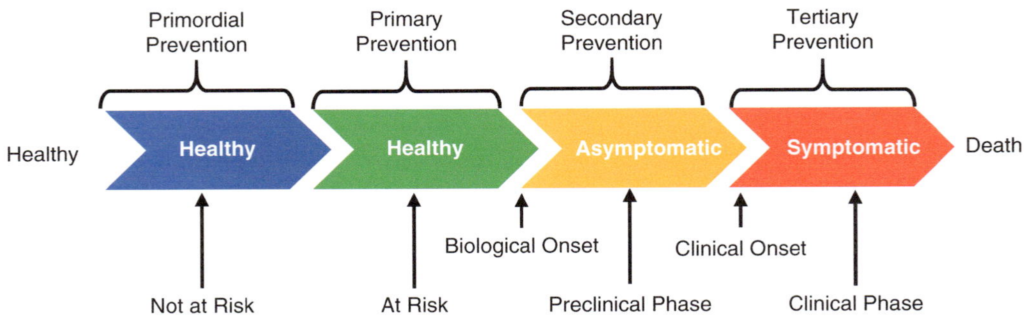

Fig. 1.1 Levels of prevention in epidemiology

reducing salt intake, encouraging physical activity, ensuring adequate sleep, and preventing childhood obesity. Additionally, addressing maternal health conditions, such as obesity and gestational diabetes, is crucial. By fostering healthy behaviors and creating supportive environments from infancy, healthcare providers and communities can help maintain normal blood pressure levels, reduce the risk of hypertension, and prevent associated cardiovascular diseases in adulthood [6].

Additional Examples

- Promoting healthy nutrition in schools to prevent childhood obesity and associated conditions such as hypertension, type 2 diabetes, and cardiovascular diseases later in life.
- Encouraging physical activity by creating safe parks, playgrounds, and community spaces to address sedentary lifestyles that contribute to obesity, high blood pressure, and cardiovascular diseases.
- Promoting breastfeeding through education and support programs for new mothers to prevent childhood obesity, infections, and chronic diseases in later life.

These actions address the *root causes* of health problems, unlike primary prevention, which targets *specific* diseases or risk factors. For example, draining swamps to control mosquitoes for malaria prevention and enhancing road safety to reduce accidents are primary prevention strategies, as they target specific diseases and risk factors.

Primary Prevention

Primary prevention involves actions designed to prevent the onset of a *specific* disease or injury before it occurs. It focuses on reducing *particular* risk factors and promoting *specific* protective measures within a population.

Examples

- Vaccination programs: Administering vaccines like the flu vaccine, HPV vaccine, or measles-mumps-rubella (MMR) vaccine to prevent infectious diseases.
- Tobacco control: Running anti-smoking campaigns and offering smoking cessation programs to prevent lung cancer, heart disease, and chronic obstructive pulmonary disease (COPD).
- Clean water initiatives: Ensuring access to clean drinking water to prevent waterborne diseases like cholera and diarrhea.
- Sanitation programs: Promoting the use of hygienic latrines and proper waste disposal to reduce the spread of infectious diseases.
- Air quality regulations: Reducing air pollution by regulating emissions from industries and vehicles to prevent respiratory diseases and cardiovascular conditions.
- Road safety laws: Enforcing seatbelt use, helmet laws, and speed limits to reduce traffic injuries and fatalities.

- Workplace safety standards: Implementing measures like protective gear and ergonomic equipment to prevent occupational injuries and illnesses.

Secondary Prevention

Secondary prevention focuses on *early* disease detection through *screening* and testing before symptoms appear, followed by timely treatment to prevent its progression to a more advanced stage.

Examples

- Mammography: Conducting regular mammograms to detect breast cancer at an early stage when treatment is more effective.
- Pap smears: Offering Pap tests to identify cervical abnormalities or precancerous changes before they develop into cervical cancer.
- Colonoscopy: Screening for colorectal cancer or polyps to enable early treatment and prevent progression to advanced stages.
- Blood pressure monitoring: Identifying hypertension early to manage it through lifestyle changes or medication, reducing the risk of stroke and heart disease.
- Diabetes screening: Testing blood glucose levels to detect prediabetes or type 2 diabetes early and initiate interventions.
- Vision screenings: Performing vision tests in children to detect amblyopia (lazy eye) early, allowing for timely treatment to prevent permanent vision impairment.
- Mental health screenings: Identifying early signs of depression, anxiety, or other mental health disorders and providing counseling or treatment to prevent severe outcomes.
- Regular dental checkups: Detecting cavities, gum disease, or oral cancer early to provide timely treatment and prevent complications.
- Prenatal care: Monitoring pregnant women for conditions like gestational diabetes or preeclampsia to ensure early management and reduce risks to mother and baby.

Tertiary Prevention

Tertiary prevention focuses on managing and reducing the impact of an already established disease. It aims to prevent *complications*, rehabilitate individuals, and improve quality of life.

Examples

- HIV/AIDS management: Providing antiretroviral therapy (ART) to reduce viral load, prevent opportunistic infections, and improve quality of life.
- Diabetes management programs: Providing insulin therapy, regular monitoring of blood sugar levels, and education to prevent complications like neuropathy, retinopathy, and cardiovascular diseases.
- Cardiac rehabilitation: Offering supervised exercise, dietary guidance, and psychological support for patients recovering from heart attacks or undergoing heart surgery to improve cardiovascular health and reduce recurrence risk.
- Chronic obstructive pulmonary disease (COPD) management: Using bronchodilators, pulmonary rehabilitation, and oxygen therapy to improve respiratory function and reduce hospitalizations.
- Stroke rehabilitation: Implementing physical therapy, occupational therapy, and speech therapy for stroke survivors to regain lost functions and improve independence.
- Spinal cord injury rehabilitation: Providing mobility aids, physical therapy, and psychological counseling to help patients adapt to life after injury.
- Prosthetic fitting and training: Assisting amputees with prosthetic devices and therapy to restore mobility and daily function.
- Dialysis for end-stage renal disease: Offering regular hemodialysis or peritoneal dialysis to manage kidney failure and prevent complications.

Conceptual Questions

1. What is the fundamental difference between primordial prevention and primary prevention? Provide examples to illustrate.
2. How does secondary prevention differ from tertiary prevention? Explain with examples.
3. Can you think of a disease or condition that could benefit from all four levels of prevention? Describe the strategies that could be implemented at each level.

1.2 Incidence Risk

Description

Incidence risk refers to the number of *new cases* of a disease that occur in a *population at risk* over a specified period of time [2, 7, 8].

A *new case* is an individual who was free of the disease at the start of the study but develops the disease during the study period.

A *population at risk* is the group of individuals who are susceptible to developing the disease. For example, women are at risk of developing uterine cancer, while men are not susceptible to it. Conversely, men are at risk of developing prostate cancer, while women are not susceptible to it [2, 8].

Example 1

The incidence risk of diabetes in a hypothetical population, as illustrated in Fig. 1.2, is the number of new cases that occur within a population at risk over the year 2024.

Formula

$$\text{Incidence risk} = \frac{\text{New cases during a specific period of time}}{\text{Population at risk during that period of time}} \times 100 = \frac{4}{20} \times 100 = 20\%$$

An incidence risk of 20% suggests that approximately 20 out of every 100 people in the hypothetical population will develop diabetes within 1 year.

The choice of multiplying the incidence risk by 100 is more or less arbitrary and can be multiplied by 1000, 10,000, 100,000, or even 1000,000.

Example 2

To illustrate the concept of incident risk, let's look an example using HIV cases. In 2021, the global population was approximately 7.9 billion [9]. The World Health Organization (WHO) reported that by the end of that year, there were 1.5 million new HIV infections [10]. Using this

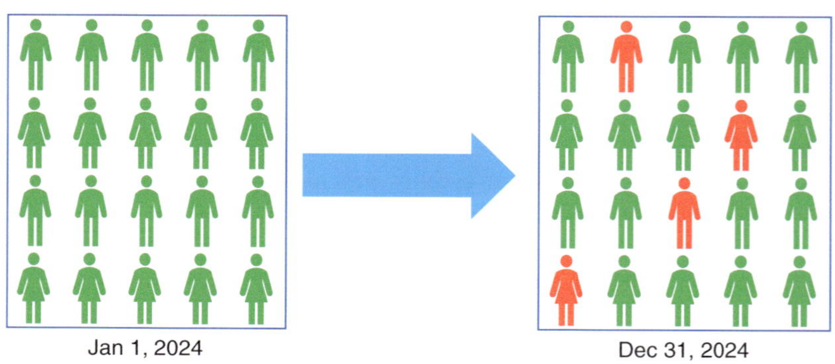

Fig. 1.2 Incidence risk of diabetes in 2024

data, we can calculate the global incidence risk of HIV in 2021 as 19.0 cases per 100,000 individuals (1,500,000/7,900,000,000).

Synonyms
Incidence risk; Incidence proportion; Cumulative incidence.

Conceptual Questions
1. What is incidence risk, and how does it differ from prevalence?
2. How can we interpret an incidence risk of 5% for a specific disease?
3. How can we calculate the number of new cases expected in a population of 10,000 individuals with an incidence risk of 2%?

1.3 Incidence Rate

Description
The incidence rate is the number of *new cases* of a disease per unit of *person-time* [2, 7, 8].

A *new case* refers to an individual who was disease-free at the beginning of the study but develops the disease during the study period.

Person-time represents the total time that susceptible participants were potentially exposed to the disease within the study, usually measured in days, months, or years.

Example 1
The incidence rate of diabetes in a hypothetical population, as shown in Fig. 1.3, is the number of new diabetes cases that occur within a population at risk, per unit of person-time.

In this example, individuals who have died or been lost during the study period are classified as lost to follow-up; however, their duration of follow-up is included in the denominator of the incidence rate. Conversely, individuals who already have the disease at the start of the study are excluded from the calculation of the incidence rate.

Formula

$$\text{Incidence rate} = \frac{\text{New cases during a specific time period}}{\text{Total person} - \text{time}} \times 100 = \frac{7}{88} \times 100 = 8\%$$

An 8% incidence rate suggests that around 8 out of every 100 people in the hypothetical population will develop diabetes each year.

The decision to multiply the incidence rate by 100 is somewhat arbitrary and could be multiplied by 1000, 10,000, 100,000, or even 1000,000.

Example 2
To demonstrate the concept of incident rate, let's consider stroke cases as an example. In the United States, approximately 795,000 new strokes occur each year [11]. This translates to an incident rate of 25 strokes per 10,000 person-years, indicating that if you observe a group of 10,000 individuals in the United States for 1 year, you can expect an average of 25 strokes to occur within that population.

Synonyms
Incidence rate; Incidence density.

Conceptual Questions
1. What is the incidence rate, and how does it differ from incidence risk?
2. How can we interpret an incidence rate of 10 cases per 1000 person-years?
3. What are the advantages of using incidence rate over incidence risk to measure disease occurrence?
4. If a study follows 1000 individuals for 5 years and 20 new cases of a disease occur, what is the incidence rate?
5. How can we calculate the number of new cases expected in a population of 10,000 person-years with an incidence rate of 5 per 1000 person-years?

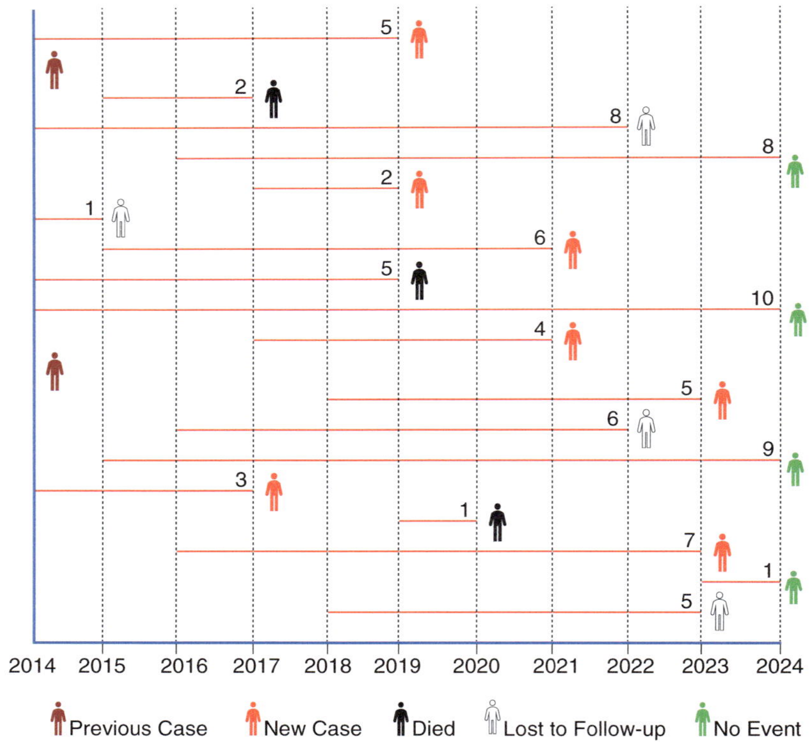

Fig. 1.3 Incidence rate of diabetes from 2014 to 2024

1.4 Point Prevalence

Description

Prevalence refers to the proportion or percentage of individuals within a population who have a specific condition at a given point in time. It highlights the total number of *existing* cases, distinguishing it from the incidence of new cases [2, 8].

Example 1

The prevalence of diabetes in a hypothetical population, as illustrated in Figs. 1.4, represents the fraction or percentage of the total population diagnosed with diabetes at a specific point in time, such as May 15, 2024.

Formula

$$\text{Point prevalence} = \frac{\text{Total existing cases at a specified time}}{\text{Total population at that time}} \times 100 = \frac{2}{12} \times 100 = 17\%$$

A 17% prevalence suggests that about 17 out of every 100 people in the hypothetical population had diabetes on May 15, 2024.

The decision to multiply the prevalence by 100 is somewhat arbitrary and could be multiplied by 1000, 10,000, 100,000, or even 1000,000.

Example 2

To illustrate the concept of point prevalence, let's examine the data on SARS-CoV-2 infections in the United States. In a random sample of Indiana residents aged 12 years and older, the estimated prevalence of present or past SARS-CoV-2 infec-

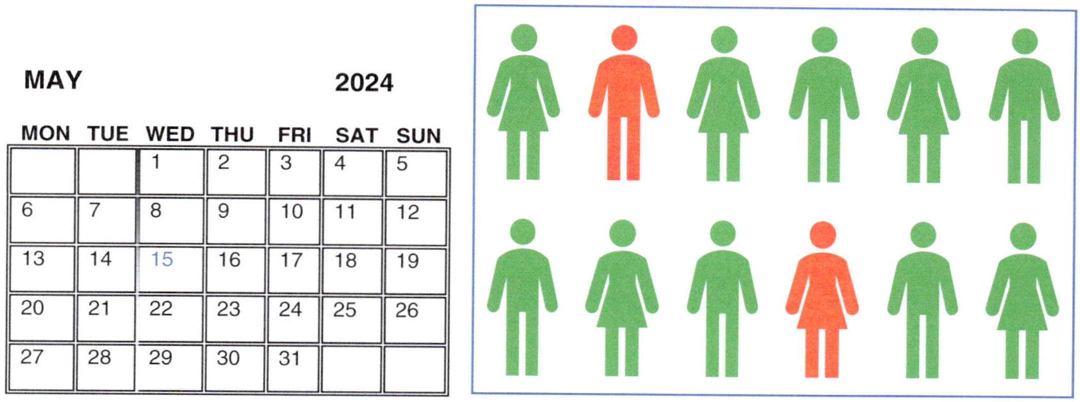

Fig. 1.4 Prevalence of diabetes on May 15, 2024

tion in late April 2020 was 2.79% [12]. This indicates that, at that time, approximately 279 individuals per 10,000 Indiana residents were infected with SARS-CoV-2.

Synonyms
Prevalence; Point prevalence; Prevalence proportion.

Conceptual Questions
1. What is prevalence, and how does it differ from incidence?
2. How can we interpret a prevalence of 25% for a specific disease?
3. If a survey of 1000 individuals finds that 200 have a certain disease, what is the prevalence?
4. How can we calculate the number of individuals with a disease in a population of 10,000 if the prevalence is 10%?

1.5 Period Prevalence

Description
The total number of individuals who had the disease at any point during the specified time period includes those who have died from it, recovered, were lost to follow-up after being affected, or are still presently affected. The key factor is that each person included in the numerator experienced the disease at some point within the designated time period, regardless of their present health status [2].

Example
The proportion or percentage of the average population with COVID-19 in a hypothetical population of 10,000 people during the year 2024, as illustrated in Fig. 1.5, includes individuals who have died from the disease, recovered, were lost to follow-up after being affected, or are still presently affected. Each horizontal line represents the duration of illness for an individual case.

Formula

$$\text{Period prevalence} = \frac{\text{All cases indentified during a specific period of time}}{\text{Average population}} = \frac{10}{10{,}000} = 0.001$$

$$\text{Average population} = \frac{\text{Baseline population} + \text{end population}}{2} = \frac{9{,}000 + 11{,}000}{2} = 10{,}000$$

Fig. 1.5 Period prevalence of COVID-19 in 2024 in a hypothetical population of 10,000 people

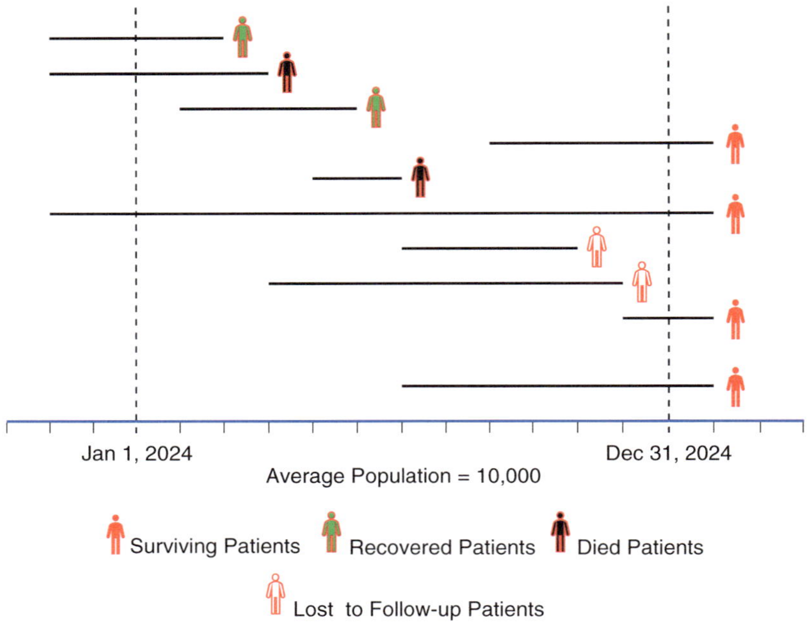

A period prevalence of 0.001 suggests that approximately one person in every 1000 individuals in the population had been affected by COVID-19 at some point during 2024, regardless of present disease status.

Conceptual Questions

1. What is the difference between period prevalence and point prevalence, and why is it important to distinguish between the two in epidemiological studies?
2. Given a period prevalence of 0.001 in a population of 10,000, how many individuals had COVID-19 at some point during the year 2024?
3. How might the status of individuals (recovered, lost to follow-up, deceased, or still affected) at the end of the period influence our understanding of the disease's impact on the community?

1.6 Herd Immunity

Description

Herd immunity, also known as *population immunity*, refers to the indirect protection from infectious diseases that occurs when a large portion of a population becomes immune. This immunity can be achieved through vaccination or prior infection. When a sufficiently high proportion of the population is immune, it creates a barrier that hinders the spread of the infectious disease from person to person, as shown in Fig. 1.6. Consequently, achieving 100% immunization rates is not always necessary for successful herd immunity. There is a specific threshold, called the *herd immunity threshold* that needs to be reached for effective protection. This threshold varies depending on the specific infectious disease and its contagiousness [2].

Example

Measles is a highly contagious disease that can cause serious complications. Before widespread vaccination, measles was very common, but thanks to vaccines, herd immunity has been achieved in many countries. This means that even if someone who is not vaccinated is exposed to measles, it is unlikely to spread widely because so many people are immune. With an R_0 estimated to be in the range of 12–18 [13], achieving herd immunity for measles requires immunizing 92–94% of the susceptible population.

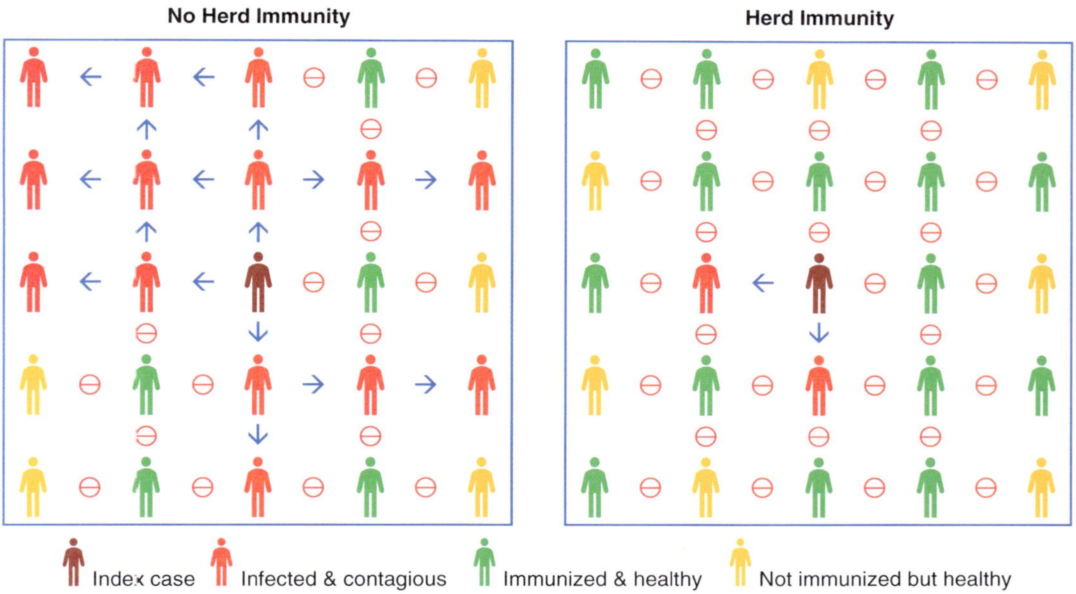

Fig. 1.6 Measles transmission with and without herd immunity

Formula

$$\text{Herd immunity threshold} = \frac{(R_0 - 1)}{R_0} \times 100 = \frac{12-1}{12} = 92\% \text{ and } \frac{18-1}{18} = 94\%$$

R_0 is the basic reproduction number. It represents the average number of secondary infections caused by a single infected individual in a population where everyone is susceptible.

Synonyms

Herd immunity; Population immunity.

Conceptual Questions

1. What is herd immunity, and why is it considered a critical concept in the management of infectious diseases like measles?
2. How does herd immunity provide indirect protection to individuals who are not vaccinated or immune? Explain the mechanism by which a high level of immunity in the population affects disease transmission.
3. Explain how the herd immunity threshold is calculated using the basic reproduction number (R_0). What does this threshold represent in terms of vaccination coverage?
4. What might happen in a community if the vaccination rate falls below the herd immunity threshold for measles?

2 Evaluating Diagnostic and Screening Tests

Contents

2.1 Validity

Description

Validity is the ability of a test to accurately distinguish between individuals *with* and *without* the disease [2]. Validity has two key components: *sensitivity* and *specificity*, as shown in Fig. 2.1.

Sensitivity is the ability of the test to correctly identify those who *have* the disease.

Specificity is the ability of the test to correctly identify those who *do not* have the disease.

	True positive: Individual actually has the disease and the test correctly shows positive.
	False negative: Individual actually has the disease, but the test incorrectly shows negative.
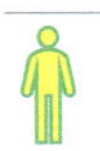	False positive: Individual does not have the disease, but the test incorrectly shows positive.
	True negative: Individual does not have the disease, and the test correctly shows negative.

Conceptual Questions

1. What does it mean for a test to have high validity? How is validity assessed in the context of medical testing?
2. Explain the significance of true positives (TP), false negatives (FN), false positives (FP), and true negatives (TN) in evaluating a test's performance. How do these metrics inform clinical decision-making?

J. Poorolajal, *Illustrated Epidemiology*, https://doi.org/10.1007/978-981-96-9566-9_2

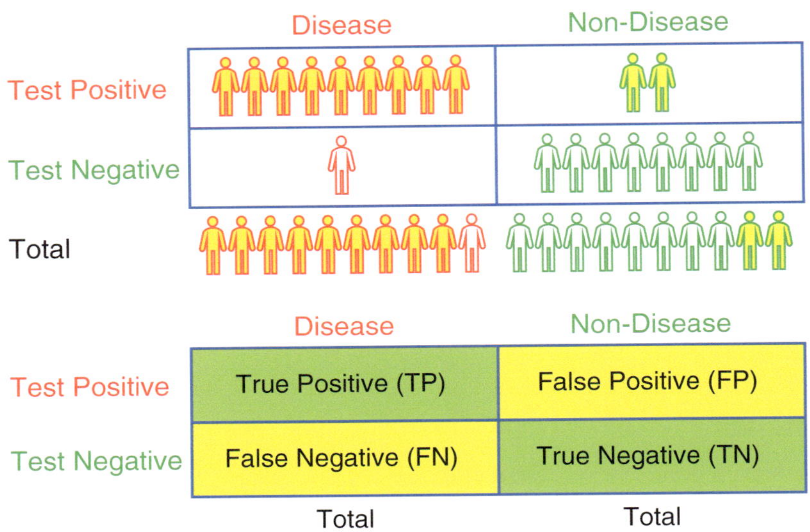

Fig. 2.1 Dichotomous test results by disease status

3. How does the relationship between true positives and false negatives affect the sensitivity of a diagnostic test?
4. What implications does the balance between true negatives and false positives have on the specificity of the test?
5. What are the potential consequences of false positives and false negatives in a clinical setting? How might these errors affect patient care and treatment outcomes?

2.2 Sensitivity and Specificity

To calculate sensitivity and specificity, a 2×2 contingency table, as shown in Table 2.1, is required.

Example 1
Consider a group of ten individuals with brain cancer. An MRI correctly identified nine of them, but one case was incorrectly negative, as illustrated in Table 2.2. Conversely, among ten individuals without brain cancer, MRI correctly identified eight as negative, but two results were incorrectly positive.

Table 2.1 Dichotomous test results by disease status

Test \ Disease	+	−
+	a	b
−	c	d
	a + c	b + d

Table 2.2 Brain cancer status classification by dichotomous MRI results

MRI \ Cancer	+	−
+	9	2
−	1	8
	10	10

Formula

$$\text{Sensitivity} = \frac{a}{a+c} \times 100 = \frac{9}{10} \times 100 = 90\%$$

$$\text{Specificity} = \frac{d}{b+d} \times 100 = \frac{8}{10} \times 100 = 80\%$$

The sensitivity of 90% indicates that the test can accurately identify 90% of individuals who have the disease. The specificity of 80% indicates that the test can accurately identify 80% of individuals who do not have the disease.

Example 2

In a case-control study evaluating the sensitivity and specificity of electrodiagnostic parameters for diagnosing carpal tunnel syndrome (CTS), researchers assessed 58 patients diagnosed with CTS and 57 control subjects without median nerve-related symptoms such as pain or paresthesia [14]. One of the primary electrodiagnostic parameters used for diagnosing CTS was the median-ulnar F-wave latency difference (FdifMU), with a cutoff value of 0.5 (≥0.5 considered positive and <0.5 considered negative). Among the 58 individuals with CTS, FdifMU accurately identified 51 cases, while seven cases were incorrectly classified as negative, as shown in Table 2.3. Conversely, among the 57 individuals without CTS, FdifMU correctly identified 53 as negative, but four results were incorrectly classified as positive.

Formula

$$\text{Sensitivity} = \frac{51}{58} \times 100 = 87.9\%$$

$$\text{Specificity} = \frac{53}{57} \times 100 = 92.9\%$$

The sensitivity of 87.9% indicates that the test accurately identifies 87.9% of individuals with CTS. Meanwhile, the specificity of 92.9% indicates that the test correctly identifies 92.9% of individuals without CTS.

Table 2.3 Carpal tunnel syndrome (CTS) classification by dichotomous median-ulnar F-wave latency difference (FdifMU)

FdifMU \ CTS	+	−
+	51	4
−	7	53
	58	57

Relationship Between Sensitivity and False Negatives

Sensitivity and false negatives are *inversely* related, meaning that as sensitivity increases, the rate of false negatives decreases. Sensitivity measures a test's ability to correctly identify individuals with a condition (true positives). A high sensitivity indicates that the test accurately identifies those with the disease, resulting in fewer false negatives. This is crucial in scenarios where early detection is vital for effective treatment.

Importantly, sensitivity and false negatives are *complementary* measures. The sum of sensitivity and the rate of false negatives equals one (or 100%), as they represent all possible outcomes for individuals with the condition.

Relationship Between Specificity and False Positives

Specificity and false positives are also *inversely* related. Specificity measures a test's ability to correctly identify individuals without a condition (true negatives). A high specificity indicates that the test accurately identifies those without the disease, resulting in fewer false positives. This is important in avoiding unnecessary anxiety, additional testing, or treatments for individuals who do not have the condition.

Similarly, the sum of specificity and the rate of false positives also equals one (or 100%). This *complementary* relationship highlights that while one metric may improve, the other may be affected, emphasizing the need for a balanced approach in diagnostic testing.

Effect of Prevalence on Sensitivity and Specificity

Sensitivity and specificity are intrinsic properties of the test and do not change with disease prevalence. They are calculated based on the test's performance regardless of how common or rare the disease is in the population.

Effect of Sample Size on Sensitivity and Specificity

Sensitivity and specificity are inherent properties of a test itself. They are calculated based on the true positive and true negative rates, which reflect the test's ability to correctly identify the presence or absence of a disease. As such, the actual values of sensitivity and specificity remain constant regardless of sample size. However, sample size does influence the reliability and precision of these estimates; larger sample sizes lead to narrower confidence intervals, enhancing the accuracy of the reported values.

Conceptual Questions

1. How do sensitivity and specificity contribute to the overall validity of a diagnostic test?
2. What is the relationship between sensitivity and specificity? Can a test be highly sensitive but not specific, or vice versa? Provide examples to illustrate your point.
3. How do sensitivity and false negatives relate to each other, and what implications does this relationship have for early disease detection?
4. What is the relationship between specificity and false positives, and why is high specificity important in clinical settings?
5. Why do sensitivity and specificity remain constant regardless of disease prevalence, and what does this mean for the interpretation of test performance in different populations?
6. How does sample size influence the reliability and precision of sensitivity and specificity estimates, and what is the relationship between sample size and confidence intervals?
7. What are the implications of having a sensitivity of 90% and a specificity of 80% for an MRI test? How should these results be interpreted in a clinical context?
8. How do sensitivity and specificity impact public health screening programs? Discuss how these metrics can affect the overall effectiveness of disease detection in populations.

2.3 Multiple Tests

Sequential (Two-Stage) Testing

In sequential testing, a less expensive, less invasive, or less uncomfortable test (Test A) is performed first. Only those who test positive on Test A are then evaluated with a more definitive test (Test B), which may be more expensive, invasive, or uncomfortable but offers greater accuracy (sensitivity and specificity). This approach minimizes *false positives*. Sequential testing decreases net sensitivity but increases net specificity, as shown in Fig. 2.2 [2].

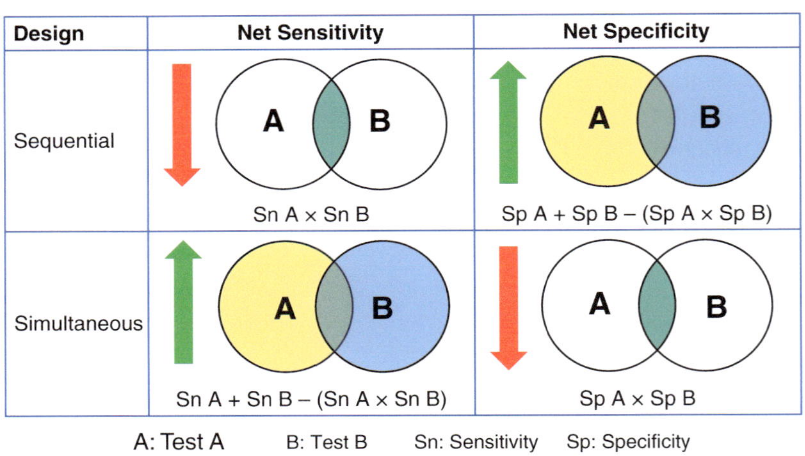

Fig. 2.2 Impact of sequential testing vs. simultaneous testing on net sensitivity and net specificity

Examples

- HIV infection: Initial screening with an ELISA test followed by a confirmatory Western blot.
- Breast cancer: Initial screening with mammography followed by a confirmatory biopsy.
- Hepatitis B: Initial screening with a rapid antigen test followed by a confirmatory enzyme immunoassay (EIA).

Simultaneous Testing

In simultaneous testing, individuals undergo both Test A and Test B at the same time. A person is considered positive if either Test A, Test B, or both tests are positive. This approach aims to minimize *false negatives*. Simultaneous testing increases net sensitivity but decreases net specificity, as illustrated in Fig. 2.2 [2].

Examples

- Tuberculosis (TB) infection: Simultaneous testing of sputum for smear microscopy and culture is a common approach in diagnosing TB.
- Heart disease: Simultaneous testing of electrocardiogram (ECG), echocardiogram, and blood tests to assess heart health.
- COVID-19 diagnosis: Simultaneous testing of PCR test and antigen test to diagnose COVID-19.

Conceptual Questions

1. What are the key differences between sequential and simultaneous testing? How does each approach affect the interpretation of test results?
2. How are net sensitivity and net specificity calculated for sequential and simultaneous testing? Explain the formulas provided in the text and their significance.
3. Discuss how the choice between sequential and simultaneous testing can impact public health strategies. How do these testing approaches affect disease surveillance and control measures in populations?

2.4 Sequential Testing

Example

Lyme disease is a bacterial infection transmitted by ticks. Table 2.4 displays the results of a hypothetical example of sequential testing for Lyme disease.

Test A: Enzyme-linked immunosorbent assay (ELISA) is a quick and inexpensive blood test that detects antibodies against Lyme disease bacteria.

$$\text{Sensitivity} = \frac{400}{500} \times 100 = 80\%$$

$$\text{Specificity} = \frac{475}{500} \times 100 = 95\%$$

Test B: Western blot is a more intricate and costly confirmatory test that examines specific antibody patterns.

$$\text{Sensitivity} = \frac{450}{500} \times 100 = 90\%$$

$$\text{Specificity} = \frac{495}{500} \times 100 = 99\%$$

A patient suspected of Lyme disease first undergoes an ELISA test. If the ELISA test is positive, the patient then undergoes a Western blot test to confirm the diagnosis.

Table 2.4 Sequential multiple testing: comparison of Test A and Test B results by disease status

	Disease	
Test A	+	–
+	400	25
–	100	475
Total	500	500

	Disease	
Test B	+	–
+	450	5
–	50	495
Total	500	500

$$\textbf{Net Sensitivity} = \text{Sensitivity A} \times \text{Sensitivity B} = 80\% \times 90\% = 72\%$$

$$\begin{aligned}\textbf{Net Specificity} &= \text{Specificity A} + \text{Specificity B} - (\text{Specificity A} \times \text{Specificity B}) \\ &= 95\% + 99\% - (95\% \times 99\%) = 99.9\%\end{aligned}$$

The confirmatory Western blot helps reduce *false positives* identified by the initial ELISA test. Sequential testing decreases net sensitivity but increases net specificity.

Conceptual Questions

1. What are the advantages of using a sequential testing approach? In what scenarios might a clinician prefer this method over simultaneous testing?
2. How does sequential testing minimize false positives while potentially decreasing net sensitivity?
3. Analyze the examples provided (HIV, breast cancer, and hepatitis B) for sequential testing. Why is a two-stage approach particularly beneficial in these cases?
4. What is the purpose of using sequential testing in the diagnosis of Lyme disease? How does this approach improve diagnostic accuracy?

2.5 Simultaneous Testing

Example

Table 2.5 displays the results of a hypothetical example of simultaneous testing used to diagnose strep throat, an infection caused by the group A *Streptococcus* bacterium.

Test A: Rapid strep test, a quick and inexpensive point-of-care test that detects specific strep A bacteria antigens from a throat swab.

$$\text{Sensitivity} = \frac{150}{200} \times 100 = 75\%$$

$$\text{Specificity} = \frac{186}{200} \times 100 = 93\%$$

Test B: Throat culture, a more accurate test where a throat swab sample is sent to a lab for bacterial growth and identification.

$$\text{Sensitivity} = \frac{184}{200} \times 100 = 92\%$$

$$\text{Specificity} = \frac{198}{200} \times 100 = 99\%$$

A patient with symptoms suggestive of strep throat undergoes both the rapid strep test (Test A) and a throat culture (Test B) at the same time. If either Test A or Test B or both tests are positive, the patient is considered to potentially have strep throat caused by the group A *Streptococcus* bacterium.

$$\begin{aligned}\textbf{Net Sensitivity} &= \text{Sensitivity A} + \text{Sensitivity B} - (\text{Sensitivity A} \times \text{Sensitivity B}) \\ &= 75\% + 92\% - (75\% \times 92\%) = 98\%\end{aligned}$$

$$\textbf{Net Specificity} = \text{Specificity A} \times \text{Specificity B} = 93\% \times 99\% = 92\%$$

Table 2.5 Simultaneous multiple testing: comparison of Test A and Test B results by disease status

	Disease	
Test A	+	–
+	150	14
–	50	186
Total	200	200

	Disease	
Test B	+	–
+	184	2
–	16	198
Total	200	200

This approach aims to minimize *false negatives*. Simultaneous testing increases net sensitivity but decreases net specificity.

Conceptual Questions

1. What are the benefits of simultaneous testing? How does this approach aim to reduce false negatives, and why is this important in certain clinical contexts?
2. Discuss the examples of simultaneous testing provided (TB, heart disease, and COVID-19). How does the simultaneous approach enhance the diagnostic process in these cases?
3. How might a clinician decide whether to use sequential or simultaneous testing for a particular condition?
4. If another diagnostic approach for strep throat were available that offered lower sensitivity but higher specificity, how might this affect the choice between simultaneous testing and the alternative method? What factors should be considered in making this decision?

2.6 Positive Predictive Value and Negative Predictive Value

Figure 2.3 illustrates the overlap between the distributions of test results for individuals with and without a disease. The area of overlap represents the potential for false positive and false negative results.

Description

Positive Predictive Value (PPV)

It is the ratio of *true positive* results to the *total* number of *positive* results (both true positives and false positives). PPV tells us how likely it is that someone with a positive test actually has the disease, as illustrated in Figure 2.4 [2].

Negative Predictive Value (NPV)

It is the ratio of *true negative* results to the *total* number of *negative* results (both true negatives and false negatives). NPV tells us how likely it is that someone with a negative test actually does not have the disease, as shown in Figure 2.4 [2].

Fig. 2.3 Distribution of true and false positives/negatives results

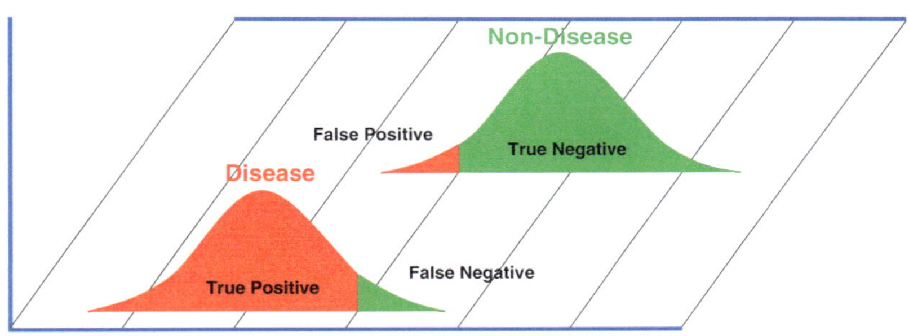

Fig. 2.4 Dichotomous test results by disease status

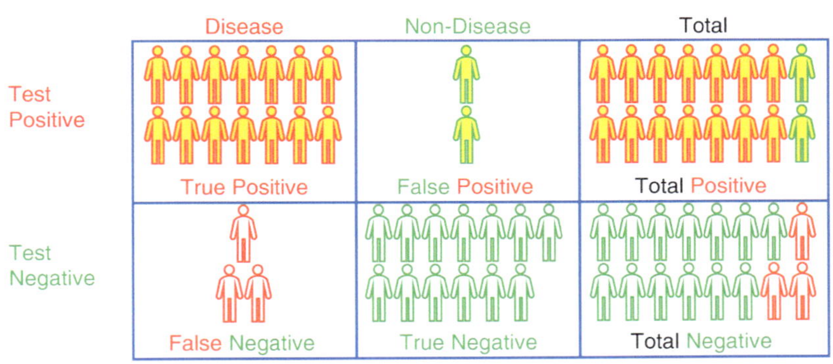

Table 2.6 Dichotomous test results by disease status

Test	Disease +	Disease −	Total
+	14 a	2 b	16 a + b
−	3 c	13 d	16 c + d

Table 2.7 Carpal tunnel syndrome (CTS) classification by dichotomous median-ulnar F-wave latency difference (FdifMU)

FdifMU	CTS +	CTS −	Total
+	51	4	55
−	7	53	60

Example 1
Table 2.6 displays a hypothetical group of 16 individuals who test positive, 14 of whom actually have the disease. Conversely, among 16 individuals who test negative, 13 are truly healthy.

Formula

$$\text{Positive predictive value}(\text{PPV}) = \frac{\text{True positive}}{\text{Total positive}} = \frac{a}{a+b} \times 100 = \frac{14}{16} \times 100 = 87\%$$

This means that 87% of individuals with a positive test result truly have the disease.

$$\text{Negative predictive value}(\text{NPV}) = \frac{\text{True negative}}{\text{Total negative}} = \frac{d}{c+d} \times 100 = \frac{13}{16} \times 100 = 81\%$$

This means that 81% of individuals with a negative test result truly do not have the disease.

Example 2
In a case-control study designed to assess the positive predictive value (PPV) and negative predictive value (NPV) of electrodiagnostic parameters for diagnosing carpal tunnel syndrome (CTS), researchers evaluated 58 patients with a confirmed diagnosis of CTS and 57 control subjects who did not exhibit median nerve-related symptoms such as pain or paresthesia [14]. One of the key electrodiagnostic parameters examined was the median-ulnar F-wave latency difference (FdifMU), which utilized a cutoff value of 0.5 (with values ≥0.5 considered positive and <0.5 considered negative), as illustrated in Table 2.7. Among the 55 individuals with positive FdifMU results, 51 were confirmed to have CTS, resulting in a PPV of 92.7%. Conversely, among the 60 individuals with negative FdifMU results, 53 were confirmed not to have CTS, yielding an NPV of 88.3%.

Formula

$$\text{Positive predictive value}(\text{PPV}) = \frac{\text{True positive}}{\text{Total positive}} = \frac{a}{a+b} \times 100 = \frac{51}{55} \times 100 = 92.7\%$$

This indicates that 92.7% of individuals with a positive test result truly had the disease (CTS).

$$\text{Negative predictive value}(\text{NPV}) = \frac{\text{True negative}}{\text{Total negative}} = \frac{d}{c+d} \times 100 = \frac{53}{60} \times 100 = 88.3\%$$

This means that 88.3% of individuals with a negative test result truly did not have the disease (CTS).

Conceptual Questions

1. What are positive predictive value (PPV) and negative predictive value (NPV)? Why are these metrics important in the context of diagnostic testing?
2. Given a test with a high PPV, what can be inferred about the likelihood that a person who tests positive actually has the disease?
3. How do false positive and false negative rates contribute to the calculation of PPV and NPV?
4. What are the potential clinical consequences of a high false positive rate in a screening test?
5. If a test has a low NPV, what does this imply about the reliability of negative test results?
6. What are the clinical implications of having a high PPV and a moderate NPV in a diagnostic test? How should clinicians use these values when making decisions about patient care?

2.7 Impact of Prevalence, Sensitivity, and Specificity on PPV and NPV

The prevalence of a disease, along with the sensitivity and specificity of a diagnostic test, significantly impacts the positive predictive value (PPV) and negative predictive value (NPV). In this discussion, we will explore various scenarios.

Table 2.8 Hypothetical scenarios of low prevalence (2%) on the left and high prevalence (20%) on the right

Test \ Disease	+	–	Total
+	18	49	67
–	2	931	933
	20	980	1000

Prevalence = 20 / 1000 = 2%
Sensitivity = 18 / 20 = 90%
Specificity = 931 / 980 = 95%
PPV = 18 / 67 = 27%
NPV = 931 / 933 = 99%

Test \ Disease	+	–	Total
+	180	40	220
–	20	760	780
	200	800	1000

Prevalence = 200 / 1000 = 20%
Sensitivity = 180 / 200 = 90%
Specificity = 760 / 800 = 95%
PPV = 180 / 220 = 82%
NPV = 760 / 780 = 97%

Table 2.9 Hypothetical scenarios of high sensitivity and low specificity (and vice versa) at high prevalence (20%)

Test \ Disease	+	–	Total
+	180	640	820
–	20	160	180
	200	800	1000

Prevalence = 200 / 1000 = 20%
Sensitivity = 180 / 200 = 90%
Specificity = 160 / 800 = 20%
PPV = 180 / 820 = 22%
NPV = 160 / 180 = 89%

Test \ Disease	+	–	Total
+	40	80	120
–	160	720	880
	200	800	1000

Prevalence = 200 / 1000 = 20%
Sensitivity = 40 / 200 = 20%
Specificity = 720 / 800 = 90%
PPV = 40 / 120 = 33%
NPV = 720 / 880 = 82%

Effect of Prevalence on PPV and NPV

As illustrated in Table 2.8, with a fixed sensitivity of 90% and specificity of 95%, an increase in disease prevalence from 2% to 20% results in a significant rise in the PPV, increasing from 27% to 82%. This trend occurs because higher prevalence indicates a greater number of true cases within the population, thereby increasing the likelihood that a positive test result corresponds to an actual case of the disease.

Conversely, in a population with low disease prevalence (e.g., 2%), most individuals tested are likely to be disease-free. As a result, a negative test result is more likely to be a true negative, leading to a high NPV of 99%. However, as prevalence increases from 2% to 20%, the number of true cases rises, which can result in a higher number of false negatives relative to true negatives. This shift results in a decrease in NPV from 99% to 97%, although the decline is not substantial.

Effect of Sensitivity and Specificity on PPV and NPV When Prevalence Is High

Table 2.9 illustrates how two different scenarios impact the PPV and NPV when disease prevalence is high (20%). The two scenarios considered are:

- Scenario 1: High sensitivity (90%) and low specificity (20%).
- Scenario 2: Low sensitivity (20%) and high specificity (90%).

In Scenario 1, where sensitivity is high at 90% but specificity is low at 20%, the PPV is relatively low at 22%, while the NPV remains high at 89%. This indicates that, despite the high sensi-

Table 2.10 Hypothetical scenarios of high sensitivity and low specificity (and vice versa) at low prevalence (2%)

Test / Disease		−	Total
	18	784	802
−	2	196	198
	20	980	1000

Prevalence = 20 / 1000 = 2%
Sensitivity = 18 / 20 = 90%
Specificity = 196 / 980 = 20%
PPV = 18 / 802 = 2%
NPV = 196 / 198 = 99%

Test / Disease		−	Total
	4	98	102
−	16	882	898
	20	980	1000

Prevalence = 20 / 1000 = 2%
Sensitivity = 4 / 20 = 20%
Specificity = 882 / 980 = 90%
PPV = 4 / 102 = 4%
NPV = 882 / 898 = 98%

tivity, the low specificity results in a considerable proportion of false positives, leading to a lower PPV.

In Scenario 2, where sensitivity is low at 20% and specificity is high at 90%, the PPV increases to 33%, but the NPV decreases to 82%. Here, the low sensitivity results in a higher number of false negatives, which negatively impacts the NPV.

These results demonstrate that when disease prevalence is high (e.g., 20%), the interplay between sensitivity and specificity influences both PPV and NPV. Notably, when either sensitivity or specificity is low, the PPV tends to be more adversely affected than the NPV in both scenarios. This underscores the critical importance of achieving an optimal balance between sensitivity and specificity to enhance predictive values in clinical practice.

Effect of Sensitivity and Specificity on PPV and NPV When Prevalence Is Low

Table 2.10 illustrates how two different scenarios impact the PPV and NPV when disease prevalence is low (2%). The two scenarios considered are:

- Scenario 1: High sensitivity (90%) and low specificity (20%).
- Scenario 2: Low sensitivity (20%) and high specificity (90%).

In Scenario 1, where sensitivity is high at 90% and specificity is low at 20%, the PPV is calculated to be 2%, while the NPV is notably high at 99%. This indicates that, despite the high sensitivity, the low specificity results in a significant proportion of false positives, leading to a low PPV.

In Scenario 2, where sensitivity is low at 20% and specificity is high at 90%, the PPV increases slightly to 4%, but the NPV decreases slightly to 98%. Here, the low sensitivity results in a higher number of false negatives, which affects the NPV, although the decline is not substantial.

These results demonstrate that when disease prevalence is low (e.g., 2%), the interplay between sensitivity and specificity significantly influences both PPV and NPV. Notably, when either sensitivity or specificity is low, the PPV tends to be more adversely affected than the NPV in both scenarios. This underscores the critical importance of achieving an optimal balance between sensitivity and specificity to enhance predictive values in clinical practice.

Table 2.11 Disease status classification by test results (sensitivity, specificity, PPV, NPV)

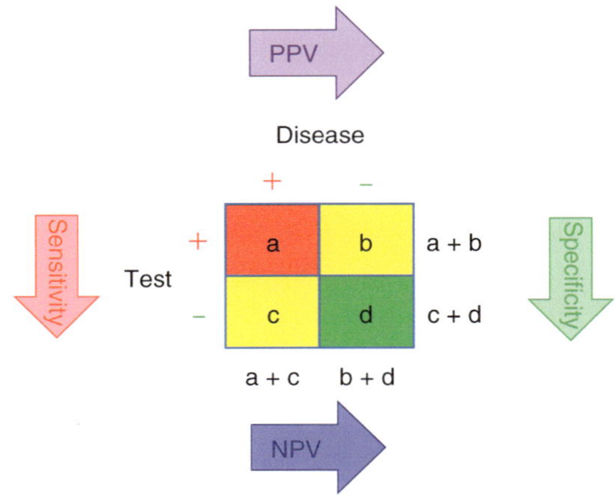

Conceptual Questions

1. How does the prevalence of a disease in a population affect the PPV and NPV of a test?
2. How do sensitivity and specificity influence PPV and NPV? Provide an example to illustrate your answer.
3. Discuss the trade-offs between sensitivity and specificity. How might a clinician decide which is more critical in a given situation?

4. Discuss how the concepts of PPV and NPV can influence public health policies, particularly in screening programs for diseases with varying prevalence rates.

2.8 Positive and Negative Predictive Values vs. Sensitivity and Specificity

Table 2.11 provides a method for calculating sensitivity, specificity, positive predictive value (PPV), and negative predictive value (NPV) using a 2 × 2 contingency table. Sensitivity and specificity are calculated by analyzing the table vertically, while PPV and NPV are derived from a horizontal analysis.

- Sensitivity is calculated as the proportion of true positives (a) among all individuals with the disease (a + c), indicating the test's ability to correctly identify those who have the disease.
- Specificity measures the proportion of true negatives (d) among all individuals without the disease (b + d), reflecting the test's capacity to accurately rule out the disease.
- PPV assesses the likelihood that a positive test result accurately indicates the presence of the disease, calculated as the proportion of true positives (a) among all positive test results (a + b).
- NPV evaluates the likelihood that a negative test result accurately indicates the absence of the disease, calculated as the proportion of true negatives (d) among all negative test results (c + d).

$$\text{Sensitivity} = \frac{a}{a+c} \times 100$$

$$\text{Specificity} = \frac{d}{b+d} \times 100$$

$$\text{Positive predictive value}(\text{PPV}) = \frac{a}{a+b} \times 100$$

$$\text{Negative predictive value}(\text{NPV}) = \frac{d}{c+d} \times 100$$

Conceptual Questions

1. Define positive predictive value (PPV), negative predictive value (NPV), sensitivity, and specificity. How do these metrics differ from one another in terms of what they measure?
2. Discuss how sensitivity and specificity relate to PPV and NPV. How can changes in sensitivity and specificity affect the PPV and NPV of a diagnostic test?
3. What are the clinical implications of understanding the differences between PPV/NPV and sensitivity/specificity? How should clinicians use these metrics when interpreting test results?

2.9 Reliability vs. Validity

Reliability

Reliability refers to the *precision* of a measurement. This means that if you repeat the same measurement multiple times, you will get similar results.

Validity

Validity refers to the *accuracy* of a measurement. This means that a measurement reflects the true value of what it is trying to assess.

As illustrated in Fig. 2.5, dartboard charts provide a visual metaphor commonly used to illustrate concepts of validity and reliability. Validity

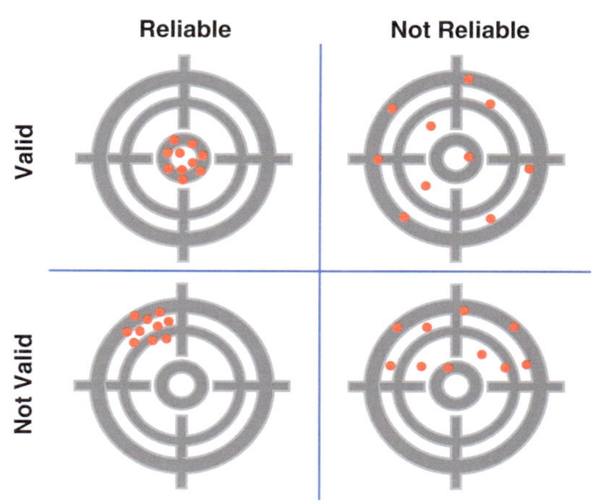

Fig. 2.5 Distinguishing validity from reliability in test results

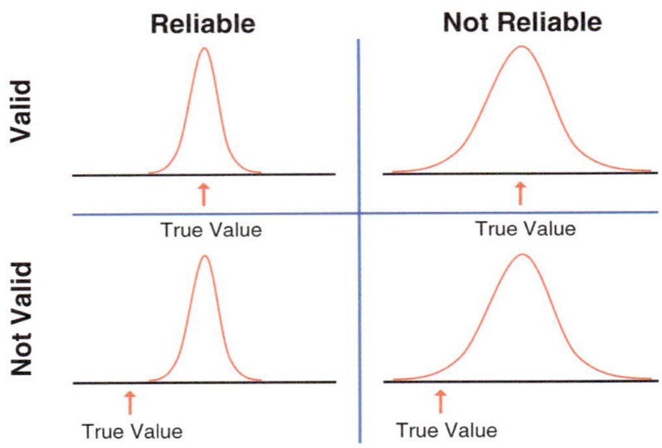

Fig. 2.6 Impact of validity and reliability on normal curve distribution

is demonstrated by how closely the darts are clustered to the center. A high degree of validity is indicated when most darts hit near the center. Conversely, low validity is shown when darts are scattered widely away from the center. Reliability is represented by how closely grouped the darts are, regardless of their proximity to the center. High reliability is indicated when the darts are clustered tightly together, even if they are not concentrated on the center. Low reliability is shown when darts are scattered widely apart.

Figure 2.6 illustrates the concepts of reliability and validity through normal curves. The width of the curve indicates reliability. A narrow curve suggests high reliability, meaning scores are consistent and clustered closely around the average. A wide curve indicates low reliability, with scores spread out more widely. The peak of the curve represents the mode, which is the most frequent score. The position of the mode in relation to the true point indicates validity. A mode close to the true value suggests high validity, meaning the measurement accurately reflects the true value. A mode far from the true value suggests low validity, indicating a systematic error or bias in the measurement.

By considering these elements, four possible scenarios can occur:

- *Reliable and valid*: A narrow curve with a mode close to the true value represents a measurement that is both *precise* and *accurate*.
- *Reliable but invalid*: A narrow curve with a mode far from the true value represents a measurement that is *precise* but *inaccurate*.
- *Unreliable but valid*: A wide curve with a mode close to the true value is less common but possible. It suggests a measure that is *imprecise* but, on average, *accurate*.
- *Unreliable and invalid*: A wide curve with a mode far from the true value represents a measurement that is both *imprecise* and *inaccurate*.

Example

Sputum smear microscopy is a common test used to diagnose tuberculosis (TB) by looking for the presence of *Mycobacterium tuberculosis* in coughed-up sputum. Here is how validity and reliability play a role.

Validity asks: Does a positive sputum smear result accurately identify the patient as having active TB, without mistaking other bacteria for TB (false positive) or missing some active TB cases, particularly in patients with low bacterial loads (false negative)?

Reliability asks: Would smears prepared from three sputum samples show the same result (positive or negative), assuming proper collection and processing techniques?

Synonyms

Reliability; Precision.
Validity, Accuracy.

Conceptual Questions

1. How do you define reliability and validity in the context of diagnostic testing? What are the key differences between the two concepts?
2. Discuss the four possible scenarios of measurement outcomes (reliable and valid, reliable but invalid, unreliable but valid, and unreliable and invalid). Provide examples of each scenario in the context of medical testing.
3. Why is validity critical in ensuring that diagnostic tests accurately reflect the true disease status of patients? What are the potential consequences of using a test that is not valid?
4. How do reliability and validity impact public health strategies, particularly in screening programs? Discuss the importance of both metrics in ensuring effective disease detection and control.

3 Epidemiological Study Designs

Contents

3.1 Classification of Epidemiological Study Designs

Description
As shown in Fig. 3.1, epidemiological study designs can be classified into two main categories: observational and interventional studies.

Observational Studies
These studies involve observing individuals and collecting data on their exposures and outcomes *without* intervening or manipulating the study environment. While they are valuable for identifying potential associations between exposures and outcomes, they cannot definitively prove causation. Observational studies can be categorized into two main types: descriptive and analytic:

- Descriptive studies typically focus on a *single* group of participants from the study population. They provide a snapshot of the group by

J. Poorolajal, *Illustrated Epidemiology*, https://doi.org/10.1007/978-981-96-9566-9_3

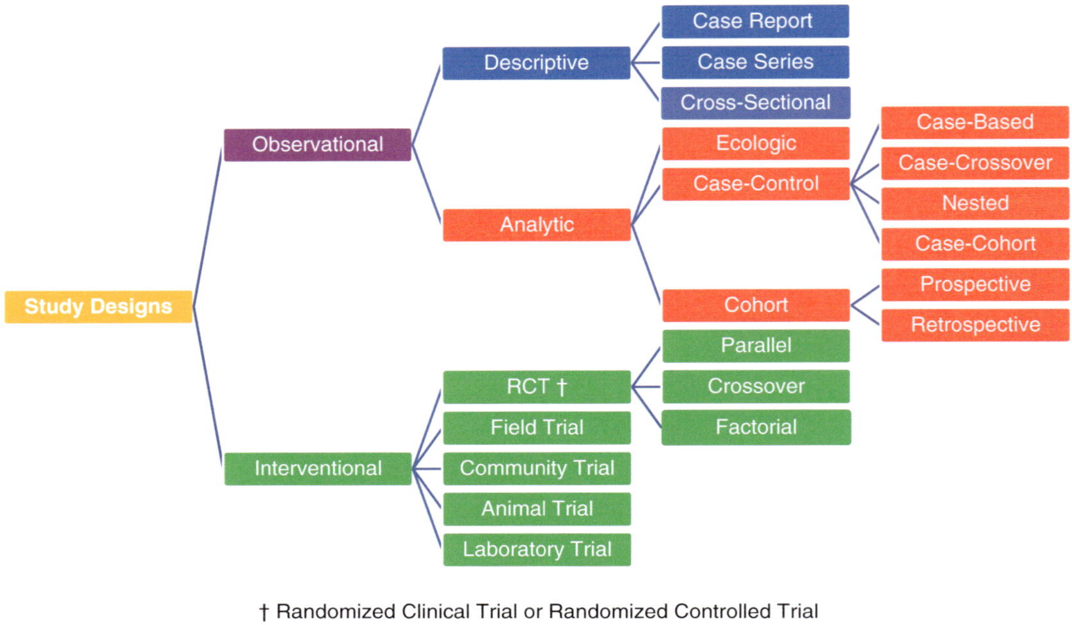

Fig. 3.1 Classification of epidemiological study designs

describing its characteristics, such as the prevalence of a disease.

- Analytic studies involve at least two *comparison* groups. By comparing these groups, researchers can investigate potential associations between exposures and outcomes.

Interventional Studies

These studies involve *manipulating* one or more variables (the intervention) in a group of participants (the intervention group) and comparing the results to a control group that does not receive the intervention. Experimental studies are considered the *gold standard* for establishing causation due to their ability to control for confounding factors. However, ethical considerations and practical limitations often restrict their applicability.

Conceptual Questions

1. What are the two main categories of epidemiological study designs? How do these categories differ in terms of their approach to data collection and analysis?
2. Define observational studies in epidemiology. What are the key characteristics that distinguish them from interventional studies?
3. What are the two main types of observational studies? Describe the purpose and methodology of each type.
4. Describe the characteristics of interventional studies in epidemiology. What distinguishes them from observational studies in terms of design and purpose?
5. What ethical considerations must researchers take into account when designing interventional studies? Provide examples of situations where these considerations might limit the feasibility of an RCT.

3.2 Case Report and Case Series

Description

Case reports and case series are methods used by healthcare professionals to document and share interesting or unusual patient experiences. However, they differ in the number of patients involved, as illustrated in Fig. 3.2.

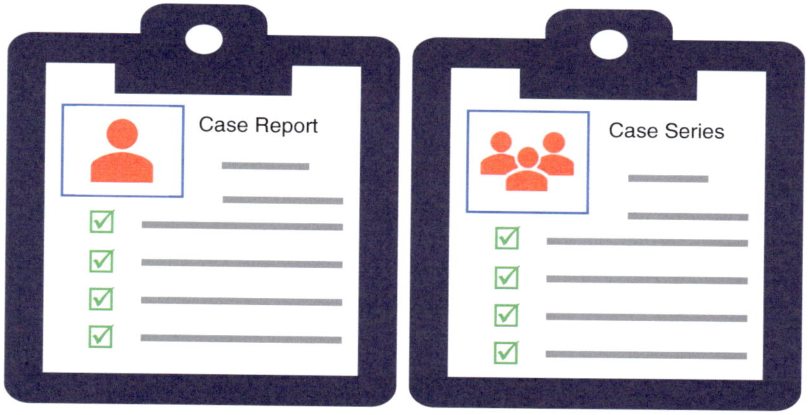

Fig. 3.2 Case report and case series designs

Case Report

A case report is a detailed description of a single individual or case. It provides an in-depth look at a patient's medical history, symptoms, diagnosis, treatment, and outcome. Case reports are often used to describe rare diseases, unusual presentations of common diseases, or special and novel approaches to disease management [2].

Case Series

A case series is a collection of individual case reports about patients with similar characteristics. These patients might share a specific diagnosis, treatment, or outcome. Case series offer a broader perspective compared to a single case report. There is no strict minimum number, but typically at least two to three patients are needed. Case series studies are observational studies that do not include a comparison group [1, 2].

Advantages

1. Detailed descriptions: Case reports and case series provide in-depth descriptions of individual cases or a group of cases, offering rich qualitative data that can highlight unique clinical features, treatment responses, or outcomes.
2. Rapid communication: They allow for quick dissemination of findings, particularly in the context of emerging health issues, rare diseases, or novel treatments, which can be crucial for clinical practice.
3. Focus on rare events: Case series can provide valuable insights into rare diseases or uncommon presentations of common diseases, which may not be captured in larger epidemiological studies.

Disadvantages

1. Lack of generalizability: Findings from case reports and case series may not be generalizable to the broader population due to the small sample size and the specific characteristics of the cases reported.
2. No control group: These studies do not include control groups, making it difficult to establish causality or assess the effectiveness of interventions compared to a baseline or alternative treatment.

Example 1

A case report described the successful pregnancy and live birth of a 45-year-old woman with recurrent implantation failure following the intrauterine administration of autologous platelet-rich plasma (PRP). After two failed in vitro fertilization (IVF) cycles and multiple embryo transfers, the patient received PRP treatment, which is rich in growth factors, administered 24 hours prior to embryo transfer. This intervention resulted in a positive pregnancy test and the delivery of a healthy baby boy weighing 2350 grams via cesarean section. This report is significant as it suggests that local administration of PRP may play a crucial role in enhancing implantation success in women with recurrent implantation failure, representing a potential new approach in assisted reproductive technology [15].

Example 2

A case report presented a rare phenomenon known as purple urine bag syndrome (PUBS), which occurs in patients with urinary tract infections (UTIs) and long-term catheterization. The report details the case of a 76-year-old female with a history of bladder cancer who developed PUBS after 4 days of constipation while hospitalized for congestive heart failure. The purple discoloration of urine, attributed to the pigments indirubin and indigo produced from tryptophan metabolism by urinary bacteria, was identified alongside a significant urinary infection caused by *Proteus mirabilis*. The patient's condition was managed with antibiotics and treatment for constipation, leading to the resolution of symptoms and discharge to a nursing facility. This case exemplifies the clinical significance of PUBS as a marker for underlying urinary infections, particularly in vulnerable populations such as the elderly with multiple comorbidities [16].

Example 3

A case series study aimed to describe the epidemiological and clinical characteristics of monkeypox in patients aged 15 and older in Buenos Aires during the outbreak from August to November 2022. A total of ten patients were included, with a mean age of 35 years: seven were men and three were women, most of whom reported engaging in risky sexual behavior. Pseudopustules were observed in 70% of the patients, all of whom had lesions in the genital, gluteal, or perianal regions. Complications included local edema, proctitis, conjunctivitis, and pharyngitis. The findings highlight the prevalence of pseudopustules as a characteristic lesion of mpox [17].

Example 4

A case series investigated the outcomes of five patients suffering from ventricular tachycardia (VT) storm refractory to drug therapy, treated with transcutaneous magnetic stimulation (TCMS) targeting the left stellate ganglion to reduce cardiac sympathetic input. The study enrolled adult patients who experienced multiple episodes of sustained VT within a 24-hour period. Following TCMS, which was administered without significant adverse events, a notable reduction in the frequency of sustained and nonsustained VT episodes was observed in the 48 hours posttreatment compared to baseline. The results suggest that TCMS may provide a noninvasive option to manage VT storm, potentially serving as a temporary solution while awaiting more definitive treatments [18].

Conceptual Questions

1. What is the primary difference between a case report and a case series in terms of the number of patients involved? How does this difference impact the type of information that can be gathered?
2. What are the main purposes of writing a case report? In what situations might healthcare professionals choose to document a case report?
3. What are some limitations of case reports and case series in terms of establishing causation or generalizability? How might these limitations affect their use in clinical practice and research?
4. How can case reports and case series serve as a basis for generating hypotheses for further research? Provide examples of how findings from these studies might lead to more extensive investigations.

3.3 Cross-Sectional Study

Description

A cross-sectional study is a type of observational research that collects data from a population at a single point in time, like taking a *snapshot* to provide information about the *prevalence* of a condition or characteristic at that moment, as illustrated in Fig. 3.3.

A cross-sectional study is typically *descriptive*, as it takes a *single* sample from the source population with the primary goal of assessing the *prevalence* of a condition or characteristic. However, it can also be *analytic* if it explores associations between variables, such as risk factors and outcomes, within subgroups of the study population.

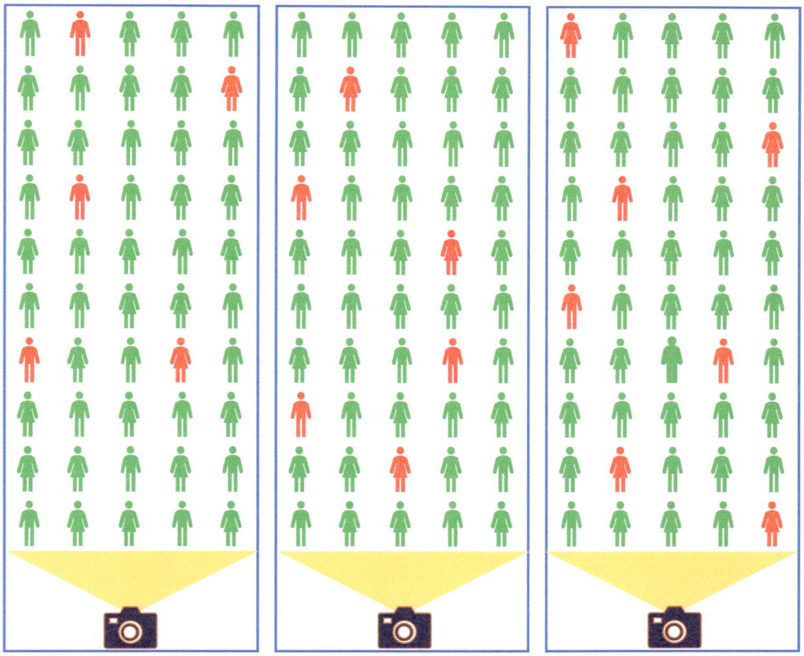

Fig. 3.3 Repeated cross-sectional studies over time (2022–2024)

Advantages

1. Simplicity and speed: Cross-sectional studies are relatively easy to design and conduct, allowing for quick data collection and analysis since they capture information at a single point in time.
2. Cost-effective: These studies are generally less expensive than longitudinal studies, as they require fewer resources and less time to complete.
3. Prevalence measurement: Cross-sectional studies are effective for measuring the prevalence of health conditions, behaviors, or risk factors within a population at a specific time.
4. Hypothesis generation: They can help generate hypotheses for further research by identifying associations between variables that can be explored in more detail in future studies.
5. Multiple outcomes: Researchers can assess multiple outcomes and exposures simultaneously, providing a comprehensive snapshot of the population's health status.

Disadvantages

1. Temporal ambiguity: The inability to assess the timing of exposure and outcome can lead to confusion about the direction of the relationship between variables.
2. Causality limitations: Cross-sectional studies cannot establish causal relationships, as they only provide a snapshot of data at one point in time, making it difficult to determine whether an exposure preceded an outcome.
3. Potential for bias: Selection bias can occur if the sample is not representative of the broader population, affecting the generalizability of the findings.
4. No change over time: Cross-sectional studies do not capture changes over time, limiting the understanding of trends or the dynamics of health conditions.

Example 1

A cross-sectional study was conducted among 4261 randomly selected Iranian university stu-

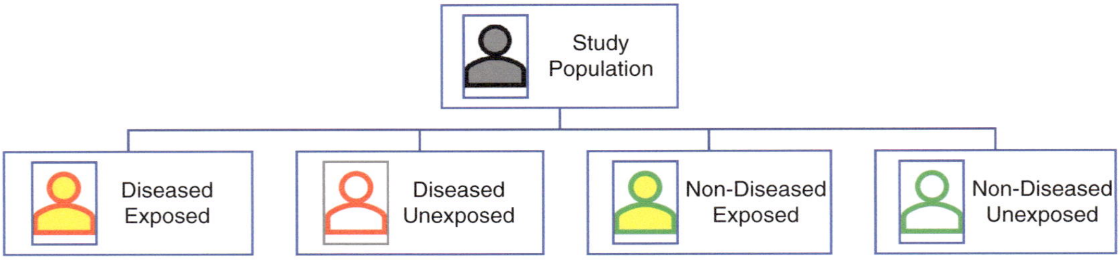

Fig. 3.4 Cross-sectional study design—identifying four subgroups based on the presence or absence of exposure and disease

dents in 2017 to determine the prevalence of problematic Internet use (PIU) disorder. Using the 15-item PIU questionnaire, the study found that approximately 27% of participants exhibited symptoms consistent with PIU. These findings provide valuable insights into the present state of PIU among this population [19].

In cross-sectional studies used for analytic purposes, both exposure and outcome variables are assessed simultaneously. As illustrated in Fig. 3.4, this approach allows for the identification of four possible groups: exposed and diseased, exposed and non-diseased, unexposed and diseased, and unexposed and non-diseased.

Example 2

Imagine a hypothetical cross-sectional study conducted to explore the link between obesity and hypertension. A total of 1000 participants were recruited and categorized as obese or nonobese based on their body mass index (BMI). Blood pressure measurements were taken to determine hypertension status. Table 3.1 summarizes this data.

$$\text{Odds ratio} = \frac{80 \times 530}{320 \times 70} = 1.9$$

The results indicate that obese individuals are 1.9 times more likely to have hypertension compared to nonobese individuals in this hypothetical cross-sectional study.

Synonyms

Cross-sectional study; Prevalence study.

Table 3.1 Obesity and hypertension—a hypothetical cross-sectional study data

		Hypertension		
		+	−	
Obesity	+	80	320	400
	−	70	530	600
		150	850	1000

Conceptual Questions

1. What is a cross-sectional study, and how does it differ from other types of epidemiological studies? What is the significance of collecting data at a single point in time?
2. What are the main objectives of conducting a cross-sectional study?
3. How do descriptive and analytic cross-sectional studies differ in terms of their goals and methods? Provide examples of each type.
4. What are some limitations of cross-sectional studies in establishing causation? Why might these studies be less effective in determining the directionality of relationships between variables?
5. What is the significance of conducting repeated cross-sectional studies over time, as illustrated in Fig. 3.3? How can this approach help researchers track changes in prevalence or associations?
6. Discuss how the findings from cross-sectional studies can influence public health policies and interventions. In what ways can these studies inform strategies for disease prevention and health promotion?

3.4 Ecologic Study

Description

An ecologic study examines the relationship between exposures and health outcomes at the *population* level rather than the *individual* level. The units of analysis in ecologic studies are typically geographically defined populations, such as countries, states, or regions, or the same population at different points in time. Average values for both the exposure and outcome of interest are calculated for each unit and compared. Visualizations, such as *scatter plots*, are commonly used to explore potential associations between the variables at the population level.

An ecologic study is typically *analytic*, examining relationships between exposures and outcomes at the group level (e.g., countries, communities). However, it can be *descriptive*, mapping the prevalence of a disease across different regions without attempting to link the disease to specific risk factors.

Ecologic studies are valuable for *generating hypotheses* and identifying potential areas for further investigation. They can also be useful for studying large-scale trends or monitoring population health. However, it is important to remember that they cannot establish cause-and-effect relationships between individual factors and health outcomes [4, 7, 8].

Example 1

As illustrated in Fig. 3.5, consider a hypothetical ecologic study examining the relationship between air pollution and asthma prevalence. Researchers might compare asthma rates across different cities with varying levels of air pollution. A positive correlation, where higher air pollution levels are associated with higher asthma rates, suggests a potential association. However, an ecologic study cannot establish causation. Other factors specific to each city, known as confounding factors, may explain the observed relationship.

Advantages

1. Cost-effective: Ecological studies are generally less expensive and quicker to conduct compared to individual-level studies, as they often use existing data from populations or groups.
2. Large sample sizes: These studies can analyze large populations, which may provide insights into trends and associations that are not easily observable in smaller samples.
3. Exploration of associations: Ecological studies are useful for generating hypotheses and exploring potential associations between exposures and outcomes at the population level.
4. Contextual factors: They allow researchers to consider the impact of environmental, social,

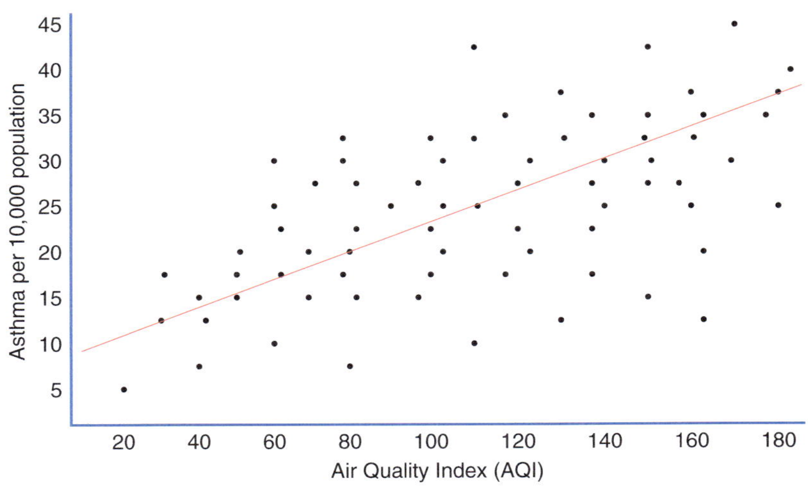

Fig. 3.5 Correlation between air quality index (AQI) and asthma cases per 10,000 population in various cities

and economic factors on health outcomes, providing a broader context for understanding health issues.
5. Feasibility: Ecological studies can be conducted when individual-level data is unavailable or difficult to obtain, making them a practical choice in certain situations.

Disadvantages

1. Ecological fallacy: One of the primary limitations is the risk of ecological fallacy, where associations observed at the group level may not hold true at the individual level, leading to misleading conclusions.
2. Inability to assess individual-level effects: These studies cannot provide information on individual-level relationships, limiting the understanding of how specific exposures affect individuals within the population.
3. Data quality issues: The reliance on existing data can lead to issues with data quality, accuracy, and completeness, which may affect the validity of the findings.
4. Temporal ambiguity: Ecological studies may struggle with establishing temporal relationships, as they often use cross-sectional data that do not clarify whether exposure preceded the outcome.

Example 2

An ecological study examined the correlation between the human development index (HDI) and the prevalence of anxiety and depressive disorders per 100,000 population across countries worldwide in 2019 [20]. The results are illustrated in Fig. 3.6. The analysis revealed a significant positive correlation between the prevalence of anxiety and depressive disorders and HDI at the global level. Notably, there was a high prevalence of anxiety and depressive disorders in countries with high and very high HDI.

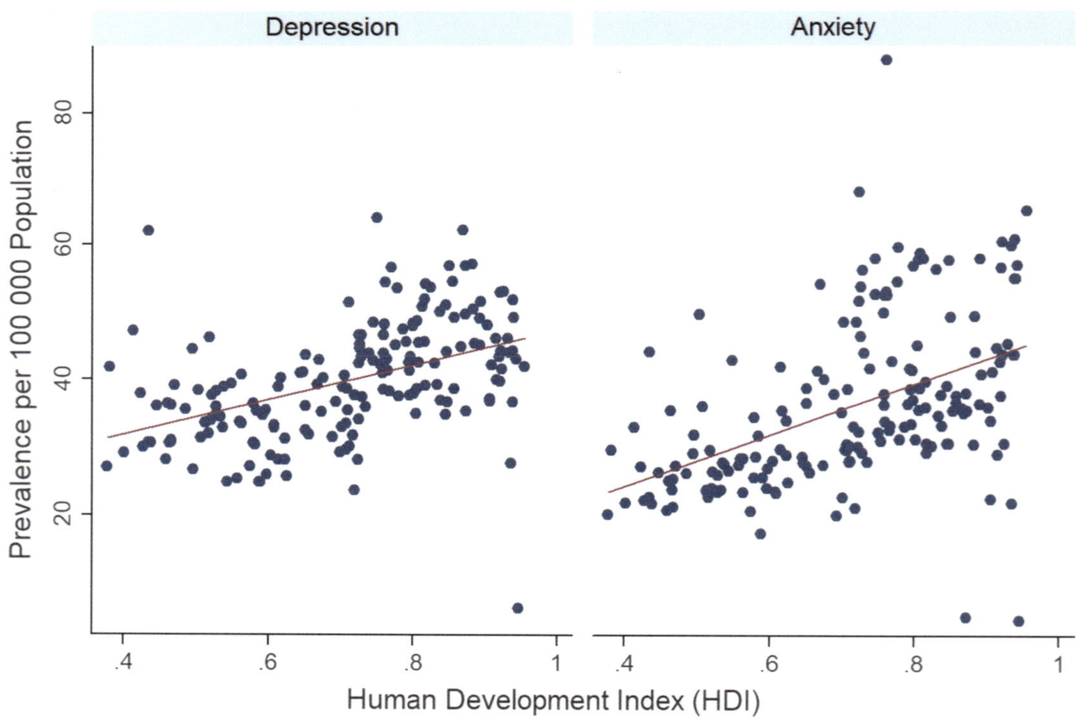

Fig. 3.6 Correlation between human development index (HDI) and prevalence of depression and anxiety disorders per 100,000 population in various countries

However, it is essential to note that a high HDI is not necessarily indicative of higher levels of depression and anxiety. This study was conducted at the country level, and many confounding factors—such as underreporting, cultural differences, socioeconomic disparities, healthcare access, and individual-level variables—were not accounted for in the analysis. Therefore, while the correlation suggests a relationship, it does not imply causation, and further research is needed to explore the complexities behind mental health trends in relation to HDI.

Ecologic Fallacy

Ecologic fallacy occurs when conclusions about *individual-level* behavior or characteristics are drawn from aggregate data for groups or populations. This type of fallacy arises because the relationships observed at the group level may not hold true at the individual level. In other words, just because a correlation exists between two variables in a population does not mean that the same correlation applies to individuals within that population.

Example 3

An intriguing paper published in *The New England Journal of Medicine* in 2012 examined the potential link between chocolate consumption and cognitive function, specifically investigating whether higher levels of chocolate consumption in a country correlate with the number of Nobel laureates per capita, which serves as a proxy for cognitive ability [21]. While a significant correlation was identified between chocolate consumption and the number of Nobel laureates across 23 countries, this analysis may be misinterpreted due to the assumption that the relationship observed at the population level applies to individuals—a classic example of ecologic fallacy. In other words, although countries with higher levels of chocolate consumption tend to have more Nobel laureates, it is fallacious to conclude that individuals who consume more chocolate are more likely to win a Nobel Prize. The correlation does not account for other factors that could influence both chocolate consumption and cognitive function, such as socioeconomic status, education, and cultural differences, which may lead to misleading conclusions about the impact of chocolate on individual cognitive abilities.

Example 4

Durkheim's ecological study of Prussian provinces from 1883 to 1890, as depicted in Fig. 3.7, demonstrates the concept of ecological fallacy. This study analyzed the relationship between the percentage of Protestants in communities and suicide rates during the late nineteenth century. By categorizing regions into four groups based on their proportion of Protestants, Durkheim estimated a rate ratio of 7.6, suggesting that suicide rates among Protestants were nearly eight times higher than those among non-Protestants.

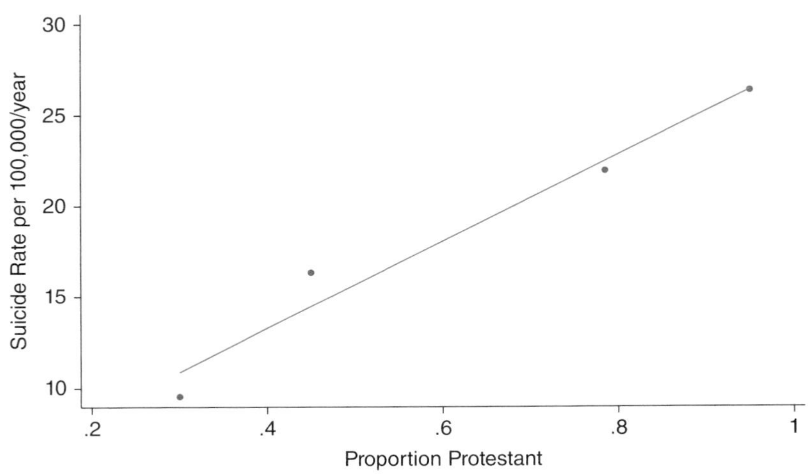

Fig. 3.7 Suicide rates by proportion of protestants in four groups of Prussian provinces (1883–1890). (Source: Adapted from Durkheim, 1951)

However, this estimate is misleading, as no region was exclusively Protestant or non-Protestant. In predominantly Protestant areas, non-Protestants (primarily Catholics) might have been at greater risk of suicide due to increased social isolation. Consequently, many suicides attributed to these areas could have been committed by Catholics, not Protestants. Durkheim's individual-level analysis, in contrast, found the suicide rate among Protestants to be only about twice that of other religious groups [22]. This discrepancy illustrates how aggregate data can mask individual-level dynamics, leading to erroneous causal inferences.

Synonyms

Ecologic study; Ecological study; Correlation study; Aggregate study.

Conceptual Questions

1. What is an ecologic study, and how does it differ from other types of epidemiological studies?
2. What are the primary units of analysis in ecologic studies?
3. What are the main objectives of conducting ecologic studies? How can they contribute to understanding population-level health trends?
4. How can ecologic studies be both analytic and descriptive? Provide examples of each type of approach within the context of ecologic studies.
5. What are some key limitations of ecologic studies in establishing causation? Why is it important to be cautious when interpreting results from these studies?
6. What is ecologic fallacy, and why is it problematic when interpreting data from group-level studies?

3.5 Case-Control Study

Description

As illustrated in Fig. 3.8, a case-control study is an observational study design used in epidemiology to investigate the relationship between a specific exposure (potential risk factor) and a health outcome (disease or condition). The study compares two groups:

Cases: Individuals who have the disease or condition of interest.

Controls: Individuals who do not have the disease.

A case-control study is inherently *analytic* due to its design. It compares cases (individuals with a specific outcome) to controls (individuals without the outcome) to identify potential associations between exposures and the outcome.

By comparing the exposure history of cases and controls, researchers can estimate the odds of developing the disease associated with the exposure, typically measured using the odds ratio, as shown in Table 3.2.

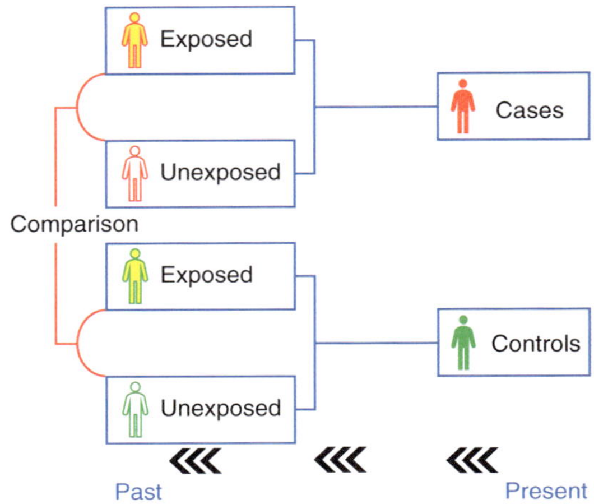

Fig. 3.8 Case-control study design

Table 3.2 Association between disease and exposure in a case-control study (2 × 2 table)

	Cases	Controls
Exposed	a	b
Unexposed	c	d
	n1	n2

Formula

$$\text{Odds ratio} = \frac{a \times d}{b \times c}$$

Advantages

1. Efficiency: Case-control studies require fewer resources and less time than cohort studies, making them suitable for studying rare diseases.
2. Cost-effective: Less expensive than cohort studies, as they do not require long-term follow-up of a large population.
3. Multiple exposures: They allow the investigation of multiple exposures in relation to a single outcome, providing a comprehensive view of risk factors.

Disadvantages

1. Recall bias: Participants, particularly in the control group, may not accurately recall past exposures, which can introduce potential bias in the data.
2. Selection bias: The way cases and controls are selected can introduce bias, affecting the validity of the results.
3. Temporal ambiguity: It can be difficult to establish a clear temporal relationship between exposure and outcome since data on exposure is collected after the outcome has occurred.

Example 1

Figure 3.9 illustrates a hypothetical case-control study investigating the association between *H. pylori* infection and stomach cancer.

- *Cases*: 500 individuals diagnosed with stomach cancer (confirmed by biopsy).
- *Controls*: 500 individuals without stomach cancer.

Both groups undergo testing to determine *H. pylori* infection status. Possible testing methods include blood tests for *H. pylori* antibodies, stool tests for *H. pylori* antigens, or gastroscopy with biopsy.

By comparing the prevalence of *H. pylori* infection between cases and controls, researchers can assess if there is a significant difference. A higher infection rate among cases suggests a potential association between *H. pylori* and stomach cancer, as shown in Table 3.3.

$$\text{Odds ratio} = \frac{200 \times 450}{50 \times 300} = 6.0$$

An odds ratio of 6.0 indicates that individuals with *H. pylori* infection are six times more likely to develop stomach cancer compared to those without the infection.

Example 2

Table 3.4 illustrates a case-control study investigating the relationship between falls and physical activity in older adults (≥60 years) [23]. The cases consist of 139 older adults who experienced a fall, while the controls include 136 older adults who did not fall in the past 3 years. By comparing the

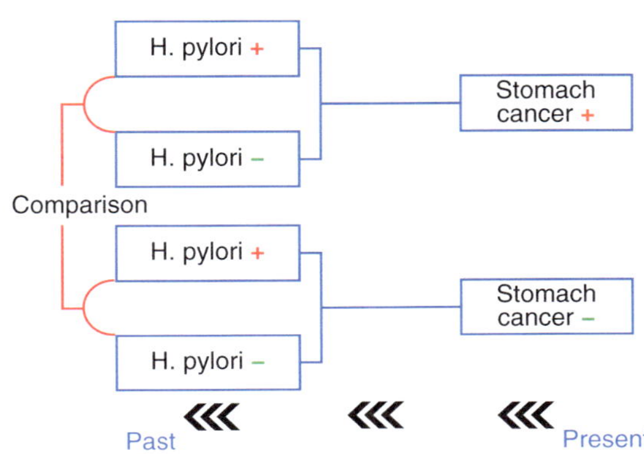

Fig. 3.9 Case-control study: *H. pylori* infection and stomach cancer

Table 3.3 *H. pylori* infection status (positive/negative) in stomach cancer cases and controls

	Stomach cancer +	Stomach cancer −
H. pylori +	200	50
H. pylori −	300	450
	500	500

Table 3.4 Relationship between falls and physical activity in older adults (≥60 years)

	Cases (falls)	Controls (no falls)
Inactive	69	59
Active	70	77
	139	136

levels of regular physical activity between cases and controls, researchers can assess whether there is a significant difference. A lower level of physical activity among cases suggests a potential association between physical activity and falls.

$$\text{Odds ratio} = \frac{69 \times 77}{59 \times 70} = 1.29$$

An odds ratio of 1.29 indicates that regularly inactive elders are 1.29 times more likely to experience falls compared to their regularly active counterparts.

Synonyms

Case-control study; Traditional case-control study; Conventional case-control study; Case-referent study; Case-based case-control.

Conceptual Questions

1. What is a case-control study, and how does it differ from other epidemiological study designs?
2. What are the primary objectives of conducting a case-control study?
3. What are the key characteristics that differentiate cases from controls in a case-control study, and why is this distinction important for the study's validity?
4. What criteria should be used to ensure that controls are comparable to cases?
5. Why is it important to establish the temporal relationship between exposure and outcome in case-control studies, and how can researchers address this challenge?
6. Explain how the odds ratio is calculated in a case-control study and what it signifies about the relationship between exposure and outcome.
7. Why is a case-control study considered an analytic study? How does it allow researchers to investigate associations between exposures and health outcomes?
8. What are some limitations of case-control studies in establishing causation? Discuss potential biases that may affect the results of these studies.
9. In what ways can recall bias affect the validity of findings in a case-control study, and what strategies might researchers employ to mitigate this bias?
10. How does selection bias arise in case-control studies, and what measures can be taken to ensure that cases and controls are appropriately matched?

3.6 Nested Case-Control Study

Description

As shown in Fig. 3.10, a nested case-control study is a variation of the case-control study that selects cases and controls from a specific population within a longitudinal cohort study. It combines key features and advantages of both cohort and case-control designs, involving the comparison of two groups: cases, who develop a particular outcome (such as a disease) within the cohort, and controls, who are cohort members that have not experienced the outcome by the time the cases do, often *matched* based on follow-up time. Notably, controls (e.g., control #2) who are at risk when each case occurs (e.g., case #2) can become cases later (e.g., case #7), allowing later cases to serve as controls for earlier ones. A nested case-control study has several advantages and disadvantages, outlined as follows [1, 8, 24, 25].

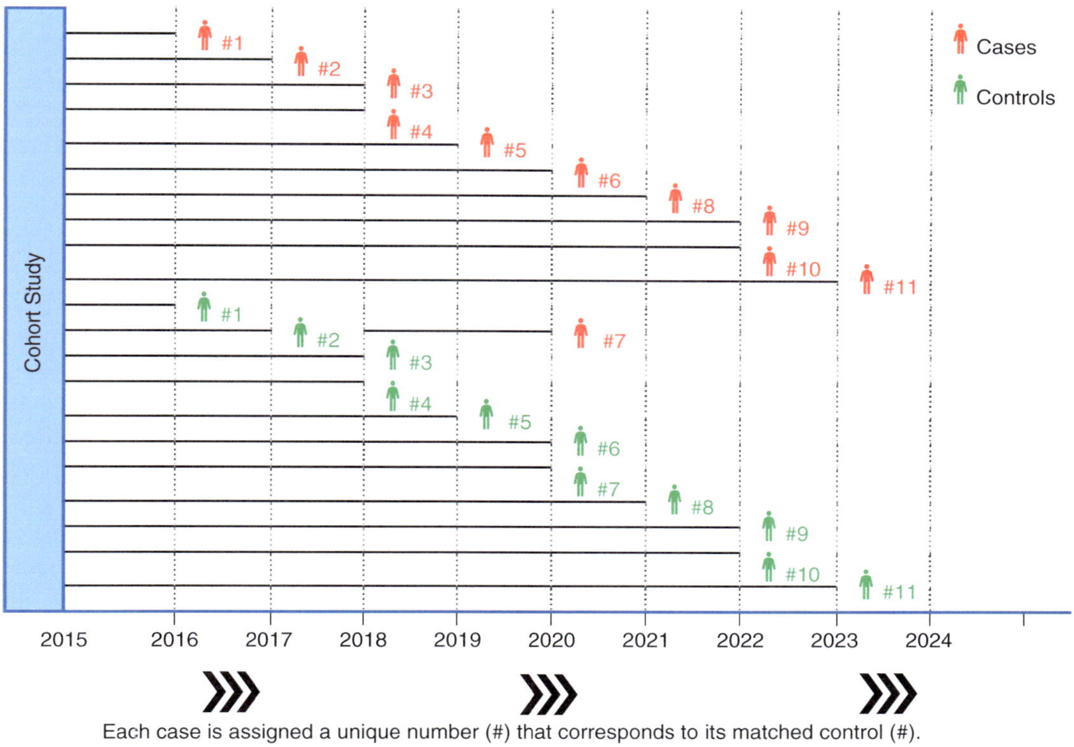

Fig. 3.10 Nested case-control study design

Advantages

1. Cost-effective: The design is particularly cost-effective when measuring exposure is expensive.
2. Reduced bias: There is a lower risk of selection bias since cases and controls are drawn from the same cohort.
3. Accurate exposure assessment: Exposure data is often collected prospectively, minimizing recall bias and leading to more accurate assessments.
4. Facilitates estimation of rate ratios: The design allows for the estimation of rate ratios, providing valuable insights into the relationship between exposure and outcomes.
5. Matching cases and controls: It enables matching based on follow-up time and other relevant characteristics, enhancing comparability between groups and further reducing bias.
6. Cost-effective for large cohorts: It allows for the efficient study of rare outcomes within a larger cohort without requiring testing of the entire population.

Disadvantages

1. Limited to existing data: The study is constrained by the data collected during the cohort study, which may not cover all relevant exposures or confounders.
2. Complexity in design: The nested case-control design can be more complex to implement and analyze than conventional case-control studies.
3. Potential for residual confounding: Although it reduces some biases, there may still be unmeasured confounders that could affect the results.

Example 1

A hypothetical nested case-control study was conducted to explore the link between the BRCA1 genetic variant and pancreatic cancer risk in a large cohort of 80,000 individuals aged

18–65 years, followed for 15 years. Blood samples were taken at the beginning and yearly thereafter. Due to the rarity of pancreatic cancer, genetic testing for the whole cohort would be expensive. Over the study period, 115 cases of pancreatic cancer were identified. For each case, four controls matched for age, sex, and smoking status were chosen. Genetic analysis for the BRCA1 variant was done solely on cases (115) and controls (460) rather than the entire cohort of 80,000. The odds ratio for pancreatic cancer risk linked to the BRCA1 variant was calculated, adjusting for potential confounders.

Example 2
In a nested case-control study within the Physicians' Health Study (PHS) [26], researchers investigated the relationship between serum markers of inflammation, such as C-reactive protein (CRP), and the risk of cardiovascular disease (CVD). The study involved 22,071 US male physicians aged 40–84 years. For each physician who experienced a confirmed myocardial infarction, stroke, or venous thrombosis (case) and had a baseline plasma sample, a control was selected from participants without CVD at the time of the event. Controls were matched to cases based on age, smoking status, and follow-up duration. A total of 543 cases and 543 controls were analyzed. The results showed that men in the highest quartile of CRP levels had a threefold increased risk of myocardial infarction (RR = 2.9, $P < 0.001$) and a twofold increased risk of ischemic stroke (RR = 1.9, $P = 0.020$) compared to those in the lowest quartile [27].

Example 3
A nested case-control study was conducted to investigate the correlation between military rank, radiation exposure, and the risk of brain tumors among male US Air Force members who had served for at least 1 year between 1970 and 1989. Researchers meticulously reviewed Air Force records to collect detailed information on radiation exposure and other relevant factors, a task that was time-consuming. To simplify the process, instead of examining the entire cohort of 880,000 individuals, researchers identified 230 cases of brain tumors and selected four race- and age-matched controls for each case, totaling 920 controls. These controls were active Air Force members at the time of diagnosis of the respective case [28].

Example 4
An 8-year nested case-control study was conducted in western Iran from April 2006 to March 2014 to investigate the risk factors associated with maternal mortality. The study included all women who had a live birth during this period. Maternal deaths that occurred within the study timeframe were classified as cases, totaling 37 cases. For each case, four women who had live births during the same period and from the same area were selected as controls, resulting in 148 controls. Conditional logistic regression analysis was performed to calculate the odds ratio (OR). The results indicated that women who gave birth at age 35 or older had more than an eightfold increased risk of maternal mortality (OR = 8.48, $P < 0.030$) compared to those who delivered at younger ages [29].

Example 5
A nested case-control study investigated the association between exposure to antidepressants and the risk of developing epilepsy using Taiwan's National Health Insurance Research Database from 1998 to 2013. The study included 863 patients with epilepsy and 3452 matched controls, categorizing antidepressant exposure based on cumulative defined daily doses (cDDD). Conditional logistic regression analysis revealed that patients with a cDDD greater than 365 had an increased risk of epilepsy (OR = 1.37) compared to those with a cDDD of less than 90. The findings suggest that long-term exposure to certain antidepressants may increase the risk of epilepsy [30].

Synonyms
Nested case-control study; Hybrid design; Ambidirectional design.

Conceptual Questions

1. What is a nested case-control study, and how does it differ from traditional case-control studies? What are the primary features that characterize this design?
2. In a nested case-control study, how are cases and controls selected from the larger cohort? What criteria are typically used to match controls to cases?
3. What are the advantages of using a nested case-control design? Discuss how this approach can improve the efficiency and validity of the study compared to a full cohort analysis.
4. How does the nested case-control study design contribute to cost-effectiveness in research, particularly when measuring expensive or time-consuming exposures?
5. Explain how nested case-control studies allow for the estimation of rate ratios. What is the significance of this capability in epidemiological research?
6. How does the design of a nested case-control study help reduce selection bias compared to conventional case-control studies, and what implications does this have for the validity of the results?
7. What advantages does the prospective collection of exposure data in nested case-control studies provide over retrospective data collection in conventional case-control studies?
8. In what ways might the limitations of existing data in a nested case-control study restrict the scope of the research, particularly regarding unmeasured confounders?

3.7 Case-Cohort Study

Description

A case-cohort study is a variation of the case-control study designed to investigate risk factors within large cohorts. In this design, researchers follow a large cohort over time, collecting baseline data on potential risk factors at the study's start. During follow-up, individuals who develop the disease of interest form the case group, while a smaller subcohort serving as the control group is randomly selected from the original cohort at baseline, which may include individuals who later become cases, as shown in Fig. 3.11. A case-cohort study presents several advantages and disadvantages, as outlined below [2, 8].

Advantages

1. Cost-effective: Exposure assessment is conducted only on a representative subcohort and all identified cases, reducing overall data collection costs.
2. Efficient use of controls: The same control group can be used for multiple cases within the same cohort, maximizing the utility of control data.
3. Estimation of risk ratios: Case-cohort studies facilitate the estimation of risk ratios, providing valuable insights into the association between exposure and outcomes.
4. Reduced bias: Since controls are drawn from the same cohort as the cases, there is a lower risk of selection bias compared to traditional case-control studies.

Disadvantages

1. Limited to predefined cohorts: The study is constrained by the initial cohort and may not account for exposures that arise outside of the predefined group.
2. Loss of information: Since only a subcohort is assessed for exposure, there may be a loss of information about exposures in the entire cohort, limiting the comprehensiveness of the analysis.

Example 1

To investigate the association between chronic *Chlamydia pneumoniae* infection and incident coronary heart disease (CHD), a case-cohort study was conducted within the Atherosclerosis Risk in Communities (ARIC) Study. Serum samples were collected from participants free of CHD at baseline, and they were followed up over a 5-year period. During this follow-up, a total of 246 cases of incident CHD were identified. The comparison group consisted of a sample of 550 participants from the total baseline cohort (referred to as a subcohort), which included 10 of

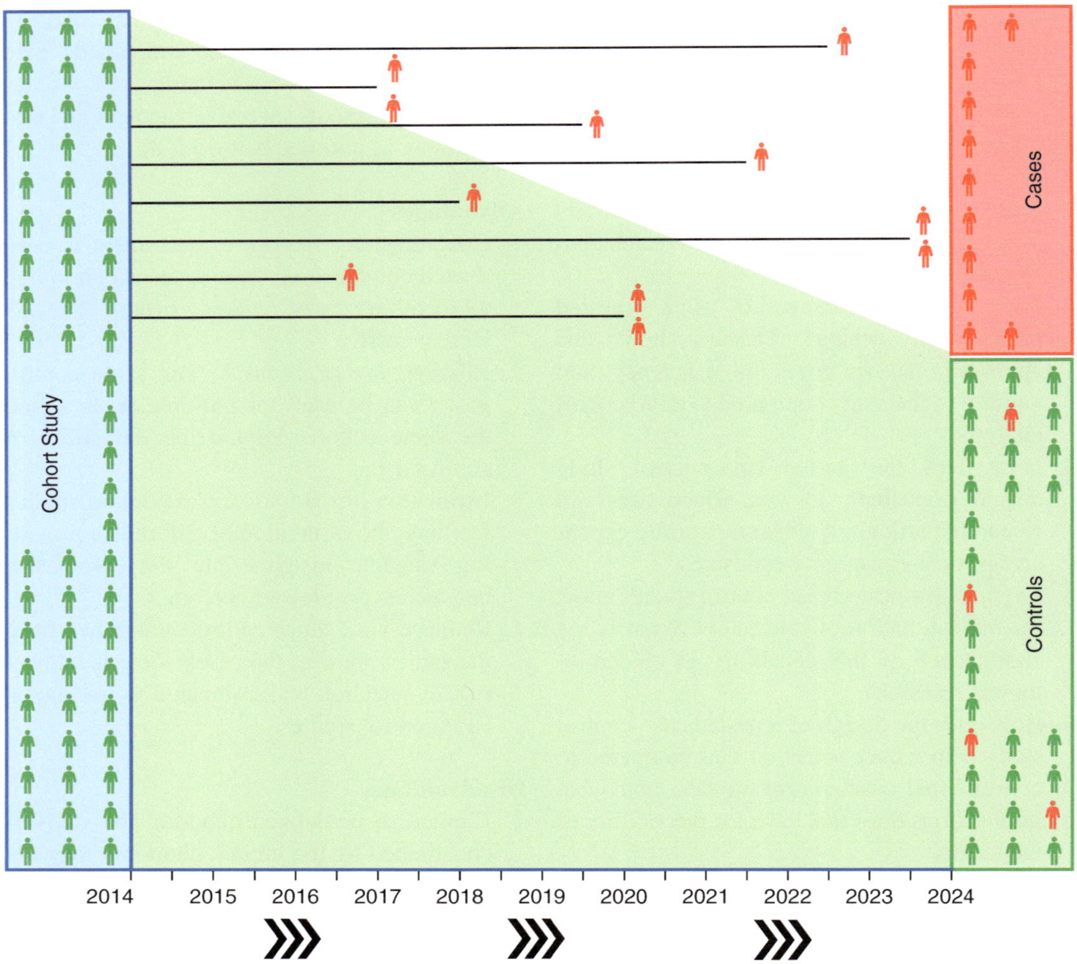

Fig. 3.11 Case-cohort study design

the 246 individuals who later developed CHD. For this study, *C. pneumoniae* IgG antibody levels were measured only in the cases and the subcohort, rather than in the approximately 15,792 cohort participants required for a full cohort analysis [31].

Example 2
A case-cohort study was conducted within the Atherosclerosis Risk in Communities (ARIC) cohort, which included 14,672 individuals aged 45 to 65. The study aimed to investigate the association between low heart rate variability (HRV) and various health outcomes. HRV was assessed at baseline using electrocardiography (ECG) records. During follow-up, researchers identified 443 all-cause deaths, 140 cardiovascular deaths, 173 cancer deaths, and 395 incident cases of coronary heart disease (CHD). A single random sample of 900 participants from the baseline cohort was selected as a comparison group for all four case groups [32].

Synonyms
Case-cohort study; Hybrid design; Ambidirectional design.

Conceptual Questions
1. What is a case-cohort study, and how does it differ from traditional case-control studies?

What are the primary characteristics that define this study design?
2. What are the advantages of using a case-cohort study design? Discuss how this design enhances efficiency and reduces costs compared to full cohort studies.
3. How does the case-cohort study design contribute to cost-effectiveness in research, particularly when assessing exposures that require extensive data collection?
4. Explain how case-cohort studies facilitate the estimation of risk ratios. What is the significance of this capability in epidemiological research?
5. In what ways does the ability to use the same control group for multiple cases enhance the validity of the findings in case-cohort studies?

3.8 Case-Crossover Study

Description

A case-crossover study is an observational epidemiological method designed to investigate the association between short-term (*acute*) exposures and abrupt (*acute*) health outcomes. In this design, individuals serve as their *own* controls. Researchers compare the exposure status of an individual during a defined period surrounding the health outcome (case period) with their exposure during one or more control periods. Choosing appropriate time windows (case and control periods) is crucial for the validity of the study. This design effectively controls for confounding factors that remain constant over the study period, such as age, sex, and genetics [2, 8, 33].

Advantages

1. Control for confounding factors: Since each subject serves as their own control, the design effectively controls for confounding factors that do not change over time, such as genetic predisposition or chronic lifestyle factors.
2. Fewer participants required: The design requires fewer participants than traditional case-control studies because each case serves as its own control.
3. Clear temporal relationship: It allows for a clear temporal relationship between exposure and outcome, as the exposure period can be precisely defined relative to the event occurrence.

Disadvantages

1. Limited applicability: This design is primarily suited for acute exposures and acute outcomes, making it less applicable for chronic diseases or long-term exposures.
2. Assumption of constant risk factors: The design assumes that the underlying risk factors are constant over time, which may not hold true in some situations, potentially leading to confounding.
3. Selection bias: There is a risk of selection bias if the cases included are not representative of the general population.
4. Complex analysis: The analysis can be more complex than traditional designs, requiring sophisticated statistical methods to account for within-subject correlations.

Example 1

Figure 3.12 represents a hypothetical study of the association between air pollution and asthma attacks, in which researchers recruited a group of individuals with asthma who had recently experienced an attack (the case). They then compared air quality data from the day before the attack (case period) with data from 2 weeks prior (control periods). As depicted in Table 3.5, by analyzing these different exposure periods, researchers could assess whether high levels of air pollution in the case period were associated with an increased risk of an asthma attack.

Table 3.6 outlines the analysis approach for matched pairs. There are three pairs (#3, #7, #10) in which both the case and the control were exposed to air pollution and one pair (#6) in which neither the case nor the control was exposed. These *concordant* pairs are excluded from the analysis of matched pairs. However, there are four pairs (#2, #5, #8, #9) in which the case was exposed to air pollution and the control was not and two pairs (#1, #4) in which the control was exposed and the case was not. These *dis-*

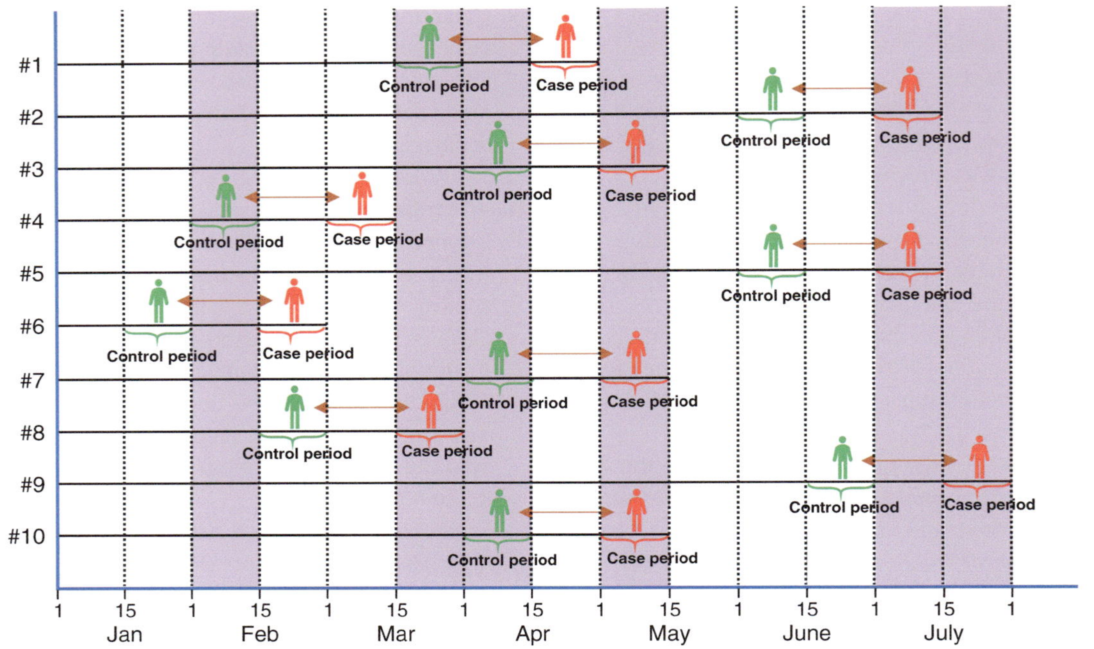

Fig. 3.12 Case-crossover study design. Colored bands indicate high air pollution periods

Table 3.5 Air pollution and asthma attacks (case-crossover study)

Cases	Controls: Air pollution +	Controls: Air pollution –
Air pollution +	a [#3, #7, #10]	b [#2, #5, #8, #9]
Air pollution –	c [#1, #4]	d [#6]

Table 3.6 Matched-pairs comparison of air pollution exposure in individuals with asthma attacks (cases) and individuals without attacks (controls)

Cases	Controls: Air pollution +	Controls: Air pollution –
Air pollution +	3 a	4 b
Air pollution –	2 c	1 d

cordant pairs are crucial for analyzing the association between air pollution and asthma attacks.

Formula

$$\text{Odd Ratio} = \frac{b}{c} = \frac{4}{2} = 2.0$$

The results of this hypothetical example suggest that people exposed to air pollution may be twice as likely to experience an asthma attack.

Example 2

A case-crossover study examined the relationship between sleep duration less than 10 hours/day and unintentional injuries in childhood, involving 292 injured children at the Children's Emergency Center in Udine, Italy. In this design, each child served as their own control; the researchers com-

Table 3.7 Matched-pairs comparison of sleep duration and unintentional injuries in children

		Controls	
		Sleeping <10 h/day	Sleeping ≥10 h/day
Cases	Sleeping <1C h/day	62 a	26 b
	Sleeping ≥1C h/day	14 c	190 d

pared the 24 hours immediately preceding the injury (case period: hours 1–24) with the 24 hours prior to that (control period: hours 25–48) [34]. The findings are presented in Table 3.7.

Formula

$$\text{Odd ratio} = \frac{b}{c} = \frac{26}{14} = 1.86\left(0.93, 3.85\right)$$

This odds ratio of 1.86 indicates that children who slept less than 10 hours per day had 1.86 times the odds of experiencing an unintentional injury compared to those who slept 10 hours or more; however, this result is not statistically significant.

Example 3

A case-crossover study investigated the link between acute alcohol consumption and injury risk among 520 injured patients in Chiang Mai, Thailand. The researchers defined the case period as the 6 hours before the injury, with control periods set for the same timeframe 1 day and 7 days prior. Findings revealed that individuals who consumed alcohol were 5.0 times more likely to be injured compared to nondrinkers, with each additional drink increasing the odds of injury by 1.3 times. The study highlighted a significant, dose-dependent relationship between alcohol consumption and various types of injuries, underscoring the need for effective strategies in Thailand to reduce alcohol-related harm [35].

Example 4

In the case-crossover study examining the relationship between temperature and infant mortality in California, researchers analyzed data from 12,356 infant deaths occurring during the warm season from May to October between 1999 and 2011. The study focused on mean daily apparent temperature, which combines temperature and humidity, and assessed its impact on all-cause mortality. Each case (infant death) was matched with control periods from the same infant, specifically using the average apparent temperature from the day of death and the previous 3 days (lag 0–3). The analysis revealed that the risk of all-cause mortality increased by 4.4% per 5.6 °C rise in temperature. The findings suggest that infants are particularly vulnerable to heat exposure, warranting further investigation in different regions [36].

Example 5

In a case-crossover study investigating risk factors for pediatric eye injuries, researchers focused on patients aged 0–18 years with severe eye trauma treated at the Canton Hospital Zenica from 2011 to 2017. The study employed a retrospective design where each case (the time of injury) was matched with two control time points: 1 month before the injury and 1 month before the survey. Out of 36 patients identified, 32 cases and 64 controls were included in the analysis. Among the various activities investigated, the results indicated that lack of supervision was associated with an odds ratio (OR) of 2.63, while sleeping less than 7 hours was linked to an OR of 4.69 for experiencing an eye injury [37].

Conceptual Questions

1. What is a case-crossover study, and how does it differ from other observational study designs? What are the primary objectives of conducting a case-crossover study?
2. Explain the concept of individuals serving as their own controls in a case-crossover study. How does this approach help to control for confounding factors?
3. Explain how the odds ratio is calculated in the context of the case-crossover study example.
4. Why is the selection of appropriate time windows for case and control periods crucial in a case-crossover study? What factors should

researchers consider when defining these periods?
5. How can findings from case-crossover studies inform public health policies and interventions? Discuss the importance of this study design in understanding short-term exposure effects on health outcomes.

3.9 Prospective Cohort Study

Description

A prospective cohort study is an observational research design that follows a group of similar individuals (referred to as a cohort) who are initially free of the outcome of interest. These individuals are followed over time to determine how variations in certain factors being studied impact the rates of a specific outcome, as illustrated in Fig. 3.13 [2, 8].

A cohort study is generally considered *analytic*, as it follows a group of individuals over time to investigate relationships between exposures and outcomes. While it can also *describe* trends within the cohort, its primary focus is on analyzing associations.

Study populations in cohort studies vary widely. They can encompass a random sample of the general population, such as the Framingham Study [38], or focus on high-risk groups like homosexual men, as exemplified by the Multicenter AIDS Cohort Study [39]. Alternatively, cohort studies might target specific populations, like the Nurses' Health Study [40] or the Health Professionals Study [41].

It is important to note that while prospective cohort studies provide strong evidence, they *cannot* definitively establish *cause-and-effect* relationships due to their observational nature. Randomized controlled trials (RCTs) are generally considered the *gold standard* for establishing causality. However, prospective cohort studies can provide valuable insights into potential associations between exposures and outcomes, as shown in Table 3.8.

Formula

$$\text{Risk ratio} = \frac{a/(a+b)}{c/(c+d)}$$

Advantages

1. Temporal sequence: Prospective cohort studies establish a clear temporal relationship between exposure and outcome, helping to understand the direction of relationships.

Table 3.8 Association between exposure and outcome in a cohort study (2 × 2 table)

	Diseased	Non-diseased	Total
Exposed	a	b	a + b
Unexposed	c	d	c + d

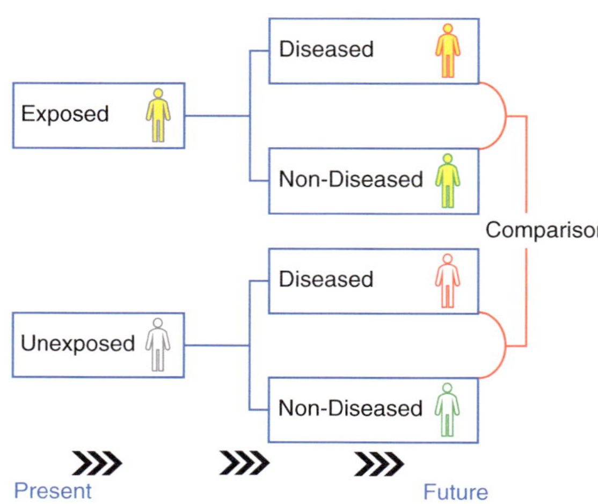

Fig. 3.13 Prospective cohort study design (present to future)

2. Reduced recall bias: Since data on exposures are collected before the outcome occurs, there is less risk of recall bias compared to retrospective studies, where participants may not accurately remember past exposures.
3. Multiple outcomes: Researchers can study multiple outcomes associated with a single exposure, providing comprehensive insights into health effects.
4. Clear definition of variables: Exposure and outcome definitions can be standardized and measured consistently, enhancing data quality.
5. Generalizability: If the cohort is representative of the general population, findings can be generalized to a broader context.

Disadvantages

1. Time-consuming: These studies often require long follow-up periods, which can take years or even decades to yield results.
2. Costly: The extensive duration and need for continuous data collection can lead to high costs in terms of funding and resources.
3. Loss to follow-up: Participants may drop out over time, which can introduce bias and affect the validity of the results if the dropouts are related to the exposure or outcome.

Example 1

Imagine a hypothetical cohort study investigating the link between smoking and lung cancer. Researchers enroll a large group of healthy middle-aged adults, collecting baseline data on smoking habits (the exposure of interest) and other relevant factors. Over many years, participants are followed to determine who develops lung cancer (the outcome of interest), as shown in Fig. 3.14.

By comparing lung cancer rates between smokers and non-smokers within this cohort, researchers can assess the potential association between smoking and lung cancer risk, as illustrated in Table 3.9.

$$\text{Risk ratio} = \frac{a/(a+b)}{c/(c+d)} = \frac{50/10{,}000}{20/10{,}000} = 2.5$$

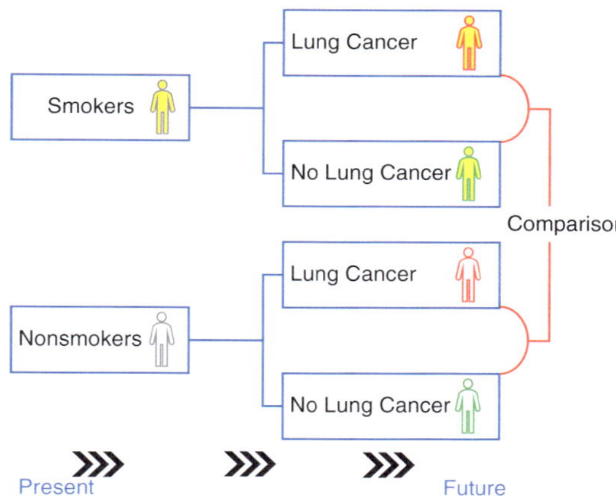

Fig. 3.14 Prospective cohort study: association between smoking and lung cancer

Table 3.9 Association between smoking and lung cancer in a cohort study (2 × 2 table)

	Diseased	Non-diseased	Total
Exposed	50	9950	10,000
Unexposed	20	9980	10,000

This hypothetical example suggests that smokers are at a 2.5 times higher risk of developing lung cancer compared to nonsmokers.

Example 2

A mixed cohort study was conducted on coronary artery bypass grafting (CABG) patients at Farshchian Heart Hospital in Hamadan, Iran, retrospectively from September 2015 to October 2017 and prospectively from October 2017 to March 2020, involving a total of 2863 patients [42]. During the follow-up period, 162 patients died, contributing to a total of 4738 person-years of observation. One of the key predictors of premature mortality investigated in this study was body mass index (BMI), with the results presented in Table 3.10.

$$\textbf{Risk ratio}_{\text{Overweight/normal weight}} = \frac{\text{Died / total}}{\text{Died / total}}$$

$$= \frac{58/1{,}199}{67/1{,}159} = 0.84$$

Table 3.10 Association between body mass index (kg/m^2) and premature mortality following coronary artery bypass grafting (CABG)

Body mass index (kg/m^2)	Died	Alive	Total	Person-years
Normal weight	67	1092	1159	1982
Overweight	58	1141	1199	1937
Obese	37	468	505	819
Total	162	2701	2863	4738

$$\textbf{Risk ratio}_{\text{Obese/normal weight}} = \frac{\text{Died / total}}{\text{Died / total}}$$

$$= \frac{37/505}{67/1{,}159} = 1.27$$

This study indicates that overweight patients have a reduced risk of premature mortality (risk ratio: 0.84) compared to normal-weight patients, whereas obese patients have an increased risk (risk ratio: 1.27) relative to normal-weight patients.

$$\textbf{Rate ratio}_{\text{Overweight/normal weight}} = \frac{\text{Died / person.years}}{\text{Died / person.years}}$$

$$= \frac{58/1{,}937}{67/1{,}982} = 0.89$$

$$\textbf{Rate ratio}_{\text{Obese/normal weight}} = \frac{\text{Died / person.years}}{\text{Died / person.years}}$$

$$= \frac{37/819}{67/1{,}982} = 1.34$$

This study suggests that overweight patients have a lower rate of premature mortality (rate ratio: 0.89) compared to normal-weight patients, while obese patients have a higher rate (rate ratio: 1.34) relative to normal-weight patients.

Example 3

A prospective cohort study was conducted to investigate the associations between metabolic syndrome (MetS) and both all-cause and cause-specific mortality, specifically focusing on heart disease, diabetes, and cancer. The study included a sample of 36,414 adults, utilizing data from the National Health and Nutrition Examination Survey (1988–2014) in the United States. Over a follow-up period of 16.71 years, a total of 8494 deaths were recorded. The findings revealed that individuals with MetS had significantly higher hazard ratios: 1.24 for all-cause mortality, 1.44 for heart disease mortality, and 5.15 for diabetes mortality. However, no significant association was observed for cancer mortality, with a hazard ratio of 1.17 [43].

Synonyms

Prospective cohort study; Concurrent cohort study; Longitudinal cohort study; Follow-up cohort study; Incidence cohort study; Forward-looking cohort study.

Conceptual Questions

1. What is a prospective cohort study, and how does it differ from other types of epidemiological studies? What are the primary objectives of conducting a prospective cohort study?
2. Why is a prospective cohort study considered an analytic study? Discuss how it allows researchers to investigate relationships between exposures and outcomes.
3. How are the risk ratio and rate ratio calculated in the context of the prospective cohort study example?
4. How does the ability to assess multiple exposures in a single study enhance our understanding of complex health outcomes, and what challenges does this present in terms of data analysis and interpretation?
5. How does loss to follow-up affect the integrity of cohort studies, and what strategies can researchers implement to minimize this issue?
6. What are the strengths of prospective cohort studies in epidemiological research? How do they contribute to understanding disease causation and risk factors?
7. What are some limitations of prospective cohort studies? Why can they provide strong evidence for associations but not definitively establish causation?

3.10 Retrospective Cohort Study

Description

A retrospective cohort study is an observational research design that examines a group of individuals (referred to as a cohort) who have been previously exposed to a certain factor (exposure) in the past. Researchers then analyze the development of a particular outcome (such as a disease or event) within this cohort by looking from the past to the present, as illustrated in Fig. 3.15. The formula for calculating the risk ratio and rate ratio is the same as in a prospective cohort study [2, 8].

Advantages

1. Time efficiency: Retrospective cohort studies utilize existing data, allowing researchers to conduct studies more quickly than prospective studies, which require long follow-up periods.
2. Cost-effective: These studies are generally less expensive since they rely on previously collected data rather than requiring new data collection.
3. Large sample sizes: Researchers can access large populations through existing records, increasing statistical power and the ability to detect associations.
4. Exploration of multiple outcomes: Similar to prospective cohort studies, retrospective studies can assess multiple outcomes related to a single exposure.

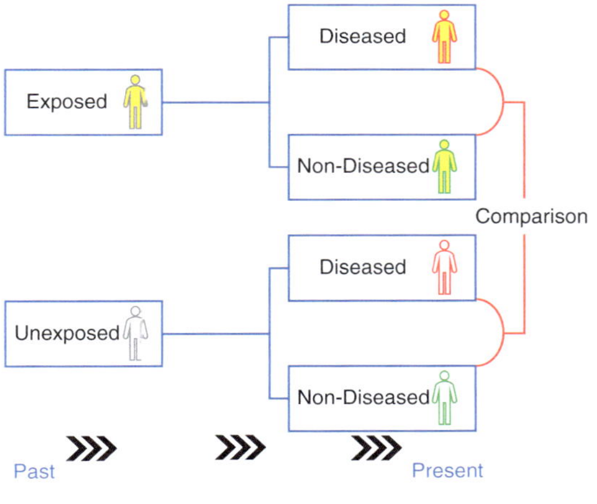

Fig. 3.15 Retrospective cohort study design (past to present)

Disadvantages

1. Incomplete data: Existing records may have missing or incomplete data, leading to potential biases and limitations in the analysis.
2. Information bias due to less control over data quality: Retrospective cohort studies often rely on existing records, where researchers have limited control over how data was originally collected. This can lead to inconsistencies or inaccuracies in the data, potentially causing information bias, where errors distort the measurement of exposures or outcomes.
3. Confounding due to unmeasured influencing factors: Since retrospective studies rely on preexisting data, they may not include all relevant variables or factors that could influence the exposure-outcome relationship. This can lead to confounding, where unmeasured or unaccounted-for variables influence both the exposure and the outcome, distorting the observed association.
4. Temporal ambiguity: Since retrospective cohort studies rely on existing data, it can be difficult to establish the correct order of events (whether the exposure occurred before the outcome). This uncertainty makes it challenging to infer causal relationships.
5. Selection bias: The way cohorts are selected from existing records may introduce selection bias, potentially affecting the generalizability of the findings.

Example 1

Table 3.11 displays the results of a hypothetical retrospective cohort study that investigated the relationship between long-term night shift work and the risk of cardiovascular disease (CVD) among retired airline pilots. Night shift work history was determined retrospectively by calculating the total flying hours between 10 PM and 6 AM throughout each pilot's career. CVD diagnoses were identified by reviewing the pilots' medical records for occurrences of heart attack, stroke, or other CVD events. Night shift work duration was classified as long-term (more than 50% of total flying hours) or short-term (50% or less of total flying hours).

Table 3.11 Risk of cardiovascular disease (CVD) by night shift work category among retired airline pilots

		With CVD	Without CVD	Total
Night shift	Long-term	72	828	900
	Short-term	20	480	500

$$\text{Risk ratio} = \frac{72/900}{20/500} = 2.0$$

This hypothetical example suggests that long-term night shift work may be associated with a twofold increased risk of CVD among retired airline pilots.

Example 2

Table 3.12 presents the results of a retrospective cohort study that investigated the association between psoriasis and the risk of all-cause dementia among patients in general practices in Germany from January 1995 to December 2014. The study compared patients diagnosed with psoriasis to those without psoriasis. The primary outcome was the cumulative incidence of dementia diagnoses over a follow-up period of up to 15 years, involving 10,583 individuals with psoriasis in the exposure group and 10,583 matched individuals without psoriasis in the comparison group. The results indicated that the incidence rates of developing dementia were 15.0 per 1000 person-years for individuals with psoriasis and 11.9 per 1000 person-years for those without psoriasis [44].

$$\text{Risk ratio} = \frac{1{,}368/91{,}031}{1{,}017/85{,}705} = \frac{0.0150}{0.0119} = 1.27$$

This result suggests that patients with psoriasis are 1.27 times more likely to develop dementia compared to those without psoriasis.

Synonyms

Retrospective cohort study; Historical cohort study; Non-concurrent cohort study.

Conceptual Questions

1. What is a retrospective cohort study, and how does it differ from prospective cohort studies? What are the primary objectives of conducting a retrospective cohort study?
2. In a retrospective cohort study, what types of data are typically collected? How do researchers access historical data to assess exposure and outcomes?
3. How does the reliance on existing records in retrospective cohort studies impact the reliability of the data, and what measures can researchers take to assess data quality?
4. How does the challenge of establishing a clear temporal relationship between exposure and outcome in retrospective studies affect the interpretation of findings regarding causality?
5. What are some limitations of retrospective cohort studies? Discuss potential biases that may affect the validity of the findings.
6. How can confounding variables impact the results of a retrospective cohort study? What strategies can researchers use to control for these confounders?
7. How can incomplete or missing data in retrospective studies affect the validity of the results, and what statistical methods can be employed to address this issue?

Table 3.12 Risk of dementia in patients with and without psoriasis (retrospective cohort study)

	With dementia	Without dementia	Total	Person-years
With psoriasis	1368	9215	10,583	91,031
Without psoriasis	1017	9566	10,583	85,705

3.11 Randomized Controlled Trial

Description

A randomized controlled trial (RCT) is considered the *gold standard* in scientific research, particularly in medicine. It is an experiment designed to minimize bias and isolate the effects of a specific intervention on a particular outcome. Participants are randomly assigned to either an experimental group or a control group, with the control group receiving either a placebo

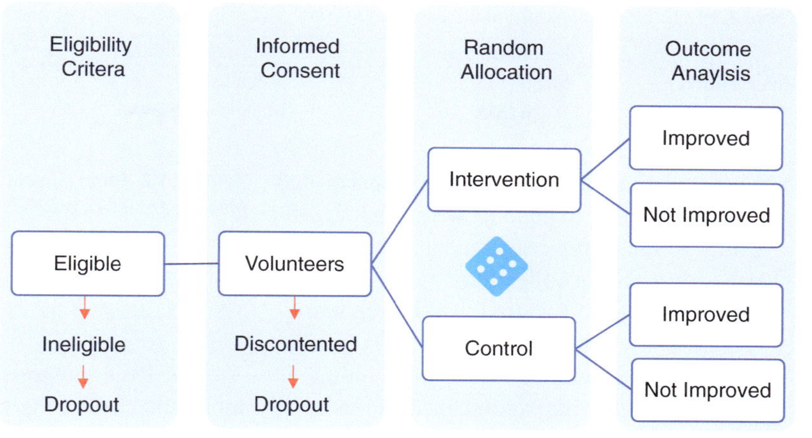

Fig. 3.16 Randomized controlled trial design

or standard treatment. As shown in Fig. 3.16, participants must meet eligibility criteria and provide informed consent before random allocation to participate in the trial. The results of an RCT with a dichotomous outcome (where there are only two possible categories) are typically presented in a table format, as illustrated in Table 3.13.

Formula

$$\text{Dichotomous outcome : risk ratio} = \frac{a/(a+b)}{c/(c+d)}$$

The results of an RCT with a continuous outcome of interest are presented in Table 3.14. This table displays the mean and standard deviation (SD) of the continuous outcome for both the intervention and control groups, measured before and after the intervention. Changes in mean outcomes for each group from before to after the intervention are calculated, followed by the determination of the differences in these changes between the intervention and control groups. This approach is known as *change score analysis*.

A more sophisticated and accurate method of analysis is *analysis of covariance* (ANCOVA), which compares post-intervention outcome data between the intervention and control groups while adjusting for baseline outcome data. This method helps control for potential confounding variables and provides a clearer understanding of the intervention's effect.

Table 3.13 2 × 2 table summarizing the intervention effect on dichotomous outcome in a randomized controlled trial

	Improved	Not improved	Total
Intervention	a	b	a + b
Control	c	d	c + d

Formula

$$\text{Change score analysis} = \text{difference1} - \text{difference2}$$

Advantages

1. Minimization of bias: Randomization helps eliminate selection bias, ensuring that participants are assigned to groups in a way that is not influenced by researchers or participants.
2. Causality: RCTs are considered the gold standard for establishing causal relationships between interventions and outcomes, as they control for confounding variables.
3. Control groups: The use of control groups allows for direct comparison between those receiving the intervention and those who do not, enhancing the validity of the results.

Disadvantages

1. Generalizability: While RCTs offer high internal validity due to their controlled design, this rigorous environment can limit external validity, making it challenging to apply the findings to broader populations or real-world contexts.

Table 3.14 Effect of intervention on a continuous outcome in a randomized controlled trial

	Before intervention	After intervention	Changes in the mean
Intervention	Mean (SD)	Mean (SD)	Difference 1
Control	Mean (SD)	Mean (SD)	Difference 2

2. Cost and time: RCTs can be expensive and time-consuming to conduct, requiring significant resources for recruitment, intervention delivery, and data collection.
3. Ethical concerns: Randomly assigning participants to a control group may raise ethical issues, particularly if the intervention is expected to provide significant benefits or if withholding treatment could cause harm.
4. Dropout rates: High dropout rates can lead to biased results and affect the integrity of the trial, particularly if the reasons for dropout are related to the intervention or outcome.

Example for Dichotomous Outcome

Researchers investigated the effect of topical furosemide compared to a placebo on the relapse chronic rhinosinusitis with nasal polyposis after endoscopic sinus surgery [45].

- Intervention group: Participants received furosemide spray, two puffs twice a day for 2 months ($n = 42$).
- Control group: Participants received placebo spray, two puffs twice a day for 2 months ($n = 42$).

Both groups continued their usual routines and medications. After 2 months, researchers compared the improvement of polyposis between the groups. The results of this RCT are presented in Table 3.15.

$$\text{Dichotomous outcome : risk ratio} = \frac{a/(a+b)}{c/(c+d)} = \frac{33/42}{16/42} = 2.1$$

Table 3.15 Improvement in polyposis in furosemide vs. placebo groups (2 × 2 RCT table)

	Improved	Not improved	Total
Furosemide	33	9	42
Placebo	16	26	42

This RCT suggests that furosemide may be more than twice as effective as a placebo in improving polyposis.

Example for Continuous Outcome

Researchers conducted an RCT to investigate the effectiveness of a vitamin D supplement in reducing blood pressure [46]. They recruited participants and randomly assigned them to two groups:

- Intervention group: Participants received the vitamin D supplement daily for 2 months ($n = 104$).
- Control group: Participants received a placebo (sugar pill) that resembled the supplement ($n = 104$).

Both groups continued taking their regular medications. After 2 months, researchers compared the changes in systolic blood pressure between the two groups. The results of this RCT are presented in Table 3.16.

$$\text{Mean difference} = 25.28 - 18.48 = 6.8(\pm 2.65)$$

This RCT discovered that vitamin D supplementation, when compared to a placebo, resulted in an average reduction of 6.8 mmHg in systolic blood pressure.

Synonyms

Randomized controlled trial; Randomized clinical trial.

Conceptual Questions

1. What is a randomized controlled trial (RCT), and why is it considered the gold standard in scientific research, particularly in medicine? What are the key features that define an RCT?
2. What are eligibility criteria in the context of an RCT, and why are they important? Discuss the process of obtaining informed consent from participants.
3. How are dichotomous outcomes different from continuous outcomes in RCTs? Provide examples of how each type of outcome is presented and analyzed.
4. Explain how risk ratios and mean differences are calculated in RCTs. What do these metrics tell us about the effectiveness of an intervention compared to a control?
5. What are the strengths of randomized controlled trials in epidemiological research? How do they contribute to establishing causality between interventions and outcomes?
6. What are some limitations of RCTs? Discuss potential ethical considerations and practical challenges that researchers may face when conducting these studies.

Table 3.16 Changes in systolic blood pressure (mmHg ±SD) following vitamin D supplementation vs. placebo in a randomized controlled trial

	Before intervention	After intervention	Mean difference
Vitamin D	152.93 (±16.42)	127.65 (±13.38)	25.28 (±18.92)
Placebo	149.45 (±14.34)	130.97 (±12.82)	18.48 (±12.98)

3.12 Crossover Trial

Description

Crossover trials are a type of clinical trial in which all participants receive the same two or more treatments sequentially. However, the order in which they receive these treatments depends on the group to which they are randomly assigned, as shown in Fig. 3.17. For example, one group might be assigned to receive treatment A followed by treatment B, with a washout period in between to allow the effects of treatment A to wear off. The duration of this washout period typically depends on the half-life of the treatment being studied.

For reliable results in crossover trials, *two* critical *assumptions* are essential:

- Short-lived treatment effects (no carryover effect): The effects of the interventions being compared must be reversible and fade away within a reasonable timeframe. This allows for a "washout period" between treatments, during which any remaining effects disappear before participants undergo the next intervention.
- Stable condition (no period effect): The underlying condition being studied should remain relatively stable throughout the trial. This implies that the condition itself should not undergo significant changes independently of the interventions. Chronic diseases or episodic conditions with predictable cycles (such as menstrual periods) are often suitable for crossover trials.

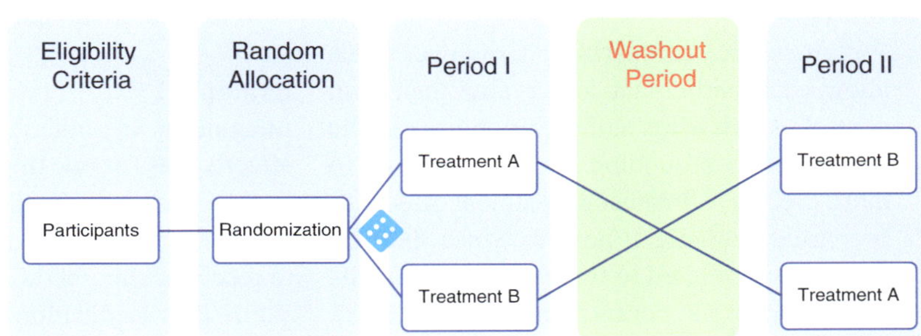

Fig. 3.17 Crossover trial design

Unlike a parallel trial where participants are randomly assigned to one group receiving only one treatment, everyone in a crossover trial receives all interventions, just in a different sequence. This way, each participant acts as their own control.

Analysis

Since each participant in a crossover trial serves as their own control, the analysis is inherently a matched analysis. When the outcome variable is continuous, the analysis typically involves comparing the means of the two conditions using a paired t-test, provided the data is normally distributed. If the normality assumption is not met, a nonparametric alternative such as the Wilcoxon signed-rank test should be employed. Additionally, researchers may consider using repeated measures ANOVA to incorporate covariates and account for within-subject variability.

For dichotomous outcomes in crossover trials, McNemar's test is the preferred analytical method, as it is specifically designed for paired nominal data. This test evaluates changes in outcomes between the two conditions, allowing researchers to determine if there is a significant difference in proportions. If the analysis necessitates adjusting for confounding variables or involves a more complex data structure, conditional logistic regression can be utilized. This approach offers a more robust analysis by accounting for the matched nature of the data and any additional covariates that may influence the outcome, thereby enhancing the validity of the findings.

Advantages

1. Within-subject comparison: Crossover trials allow each participant to serve as their own control, which helps reduce variability and the impact of confounding factors, leading to more precise estimates of treatment effects.
2. Increased statistical power: Since participants are compared to themselves across different treatment periods, crossover designs often require fewer participants than parallel-group designs to achieve the same statistical power.

Disadvantages

1. Not applicable for short-term diseases: Crossover trials may not be suitable for short-term diseases or acute conditions, where the timing of treatment and the rapid progression of the disease can limit the ability to switch treatments effectively.
2. Not suitable for all interventions: Crossover designs may not be appropriate for interventions with long-lasting effects or treatments that fundamentally alter the condition being studied.
3. Period effects: Changes in participants' responses over time (period effects) can influence the results, particularly if external factors or changes in the participants' condition occur during the trial.
4. Carryover effects: One of the main challenges is the potential for carryover effects, where the effects of the first treatment persist into the second treatment period, complicating the interpretation of results.
5. Washout periods: To minimize carryover effects, adequate washout periods are required between treatments, which can lengthen the duration of the trial and may not be feasible for all interventions.
6. Participant dropout: If participants drop out during the trial, it can complicate the analysis and affect the validity of the results, particularly if dropout is related to the treatment received.
7. Complexity in design and analysis: Crossover trials can be more complex to design and analyze, requiring careful consideration of the order of treatments and potential biases related to treatment sequence.

Example 1

Imagine a hypothetical study comparing the effectiveness of two different pain relievers, medication A and medication B. In a crossover trial design, participants would be randomly assigned to receive either medication A followed by medication B or medication B followed by medication A. A washout period would be included between treatments to ensure that any effects from the first medication wear off before starting the second.

The main outcome, pain relief, is measured using the visual analog scale (VAS). By the end of the study, researchers can compare the pain relief experienced by participants for both medications.

To analyze the results of the crossover trial, the mean VAS score for pain relief after receiving medication A is compared to the mean score after receiving medication B. This comparison allows researchers to assess the effectiveness of each medication in alleviating pain, as illustrated in Table 3.17.

Example 2

Crossover trials can be conducted with multiple treatments and periods, as illustrated in Fig. 3.18. In this specific example, researchers investigated the impact of mint, mefenamic acid, and a placebo on dysmenorrhea in young adult female students over 3 consecutive months [47].

To analyze the results of this crossover trial, researchers compared the mean visual analog scale (VAS) score for each treatment across all three periods (P1, P2, and P3). This comparison between each treatment and the other two was performed using paired t-tests.

- *Mint vs. mefenamic acid*: Mean effect of mint – mean effect of mefenamic acid.
- *Mint vs. placebo*: Mean effect of mint – mean effect of placebo.
- *Mefenamic acid vs. placebo*: Mean effect of mefenamic acid – mean effect of placebo.

Conceptual Questions

1. What is a crossover trial, and how does it differ from parallel clinical trial designs? What are the key characteristics that define a crossover trial?
2. Explain the purpose of a washout period in a crossover trial. Why is it important to allow sufficient time for the effects of the first treatment to dissipate before administering the second treatment?
3. Discuss how crossover trials can be adapted to evaluate multiple treatments. What considerations must researchers keep in mind when designing a trial with more than two treatments?
4. Why is it essential for the underlying condition being studied to remain stable throughout a

Table 3.17 Statistical analysis of crossover trial results

Groups	Period 1		Period 2	Outcome analysis
Group 1	Medication A_1	Washout	Medication B_2	Mean $(A_1 + A_2)$ – mean $(B_1 + B_2)$
Group 2	Medication B_1		Medication A_2	

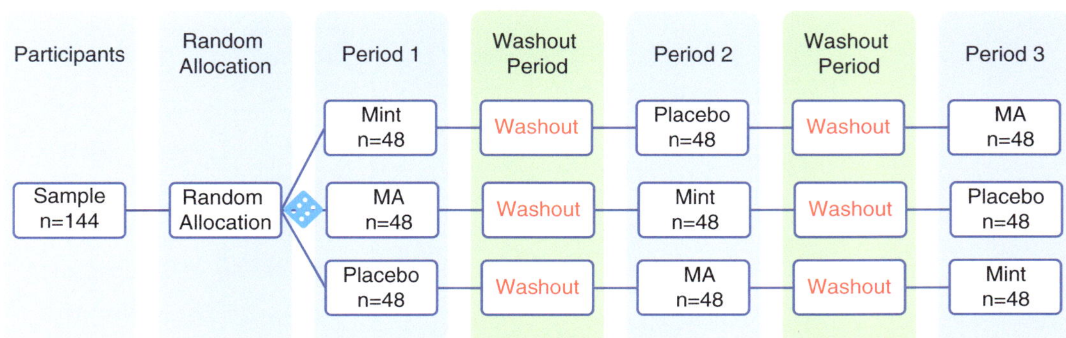

Fig. 3.18 Crossover trial design: evaluating mint, mefenamic acid (MA), and placebo for dysmenorrhea

crossover trial? How might fluctuations in the condition affect the validity of the trial results?
5. What are period effects and carryover effects in the context of crossover trials? How can these effects confound the results, and what strategies can researchers use to minimize their impact?

3.13 Factorial Trial

Description
A factorial trial design is a type of clinical trial that evaluates the effects of multiple interventions (factors) simultaneously by randomly assigning participants to various combinations of these interventions, as illustrated in Fig. 3.19. This approach enables researchers to isolate the individual effects of each factor, as well as the combined effects and potential interactions between them. By combining multiple comparisons into a single study, factorial designs require fewer participants and have the potential to save time and resources.

Analysis
In factorial trial designs, as shown in Table 3.18, if the effects of the two treatments are truly independent (no interaction), we can evaluate the effect of treatment A on outcome 1 by simply comparing participants who received treatment A (left column) with those who did not (right column). Similarly, the effect of treatment B on outcome 2 can be assessed by comparing participants who received treatment B (upper row) with those who did not (lower row).

Advantages
1. Less participants required: By studying multiple factors at once, factorial designs can often require fewer participants than conducting separate trials for each intervention.
2. Efficiency: Factorial designs allow researchers to evaluate multiple interventions or treatment combinations simultaneously within a single study, making the most efficient use of resources and time.
3. Interactions assessment: These trials enable the examination of interactions between treatments, providing insights into how different interventions may work together or affect each other.

Disadvantages
1. Participants must have both outcomes: In factorial designs, participants are typically required to have both outcomes of interest. This requirement can complicate the recruitment process, making it more challenging to identify eligible participants.
2. Complexity: The design and analysis of factorial trials can be complex, requiring careful

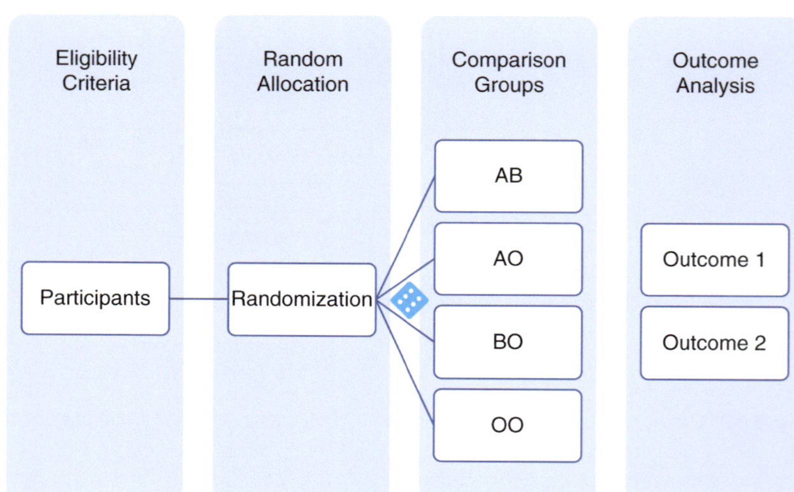

Fig. 3.19 Factorial trial design

Table 3.18 Factorial design for examining the effects of two treatments

		Treatment A +	Treatment A −
Treatment B	+	AB	BO
Treatment B	−	AO	OO

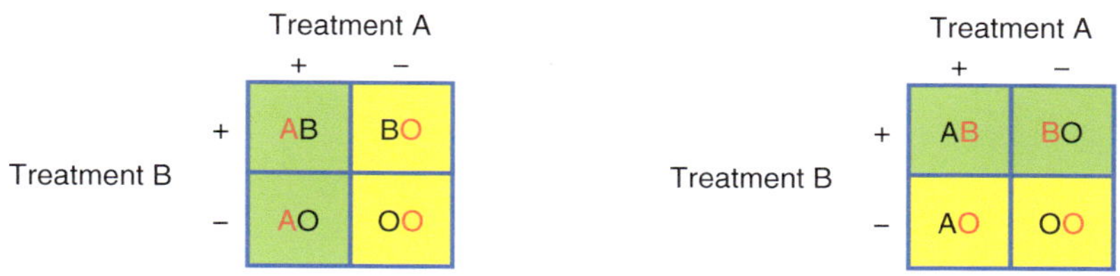

planning to ensure that all combinations are adequately represented and that the results are interpretable.

3. Potential for confounding: If not properly controlled, interactions between treatments can lead to confounding variables that complicate the interpretation of results.

Example

Researchers conducted a factorial trial design to investigate the impact of aspirin on the primary prevention of cardiovascular disease (CVD) and beta-carotene on the primary prevention of cancer [48]. They enrolled 22,071 male physicians and randomly assigned them to receive one of four possible interventions: (a) both aspirin and beta-carotene, (b) aspirin and placebo, (c) beta-carotene and placebo, and (d) neither aspirin nor beta-carotene. The resulting four groups are shown in Figs. 3.20 and 3.21.

In factorial trial designs, as shown in Table 3.19, if the effects of aspirin and beta-carotene are truly independent, we can evaluate the impact of aspirin on the prevention of cardiovascular disease (CVD) by comparing participants who received aspirin (left column) with those who did not (right column). Similarly, we can evaluate the impact of beta-carotene on the primary prevention of cancer by comparing participants who received beta-carotene (upper row) with those who did not (lower row).

Conceptual Questions

1. What is a factorial trial, and how does it differ from other clinical trial designs? What are the primary objectives of conducting a factorial trial?
2. Explain how factorial trials allow researchers to isolate the individual effects of each intervention. What does it mean for the effects to be independent, and why is this assumption important?
3. What are the potential benefits of assessing combined effects in a factorial trial? How can understanding interactions between treatments enhance the interpretation of the results?
4. Discuss how factorial trial designs can save time and resources compared to conducting separate trials for each intervention. What are the advantages of combining multiple comparisons into a single study?
5. What are some limitations of factorial trials? Discuss potential challenges related to the complexity of the design and the interpretation of interactions between treatments.

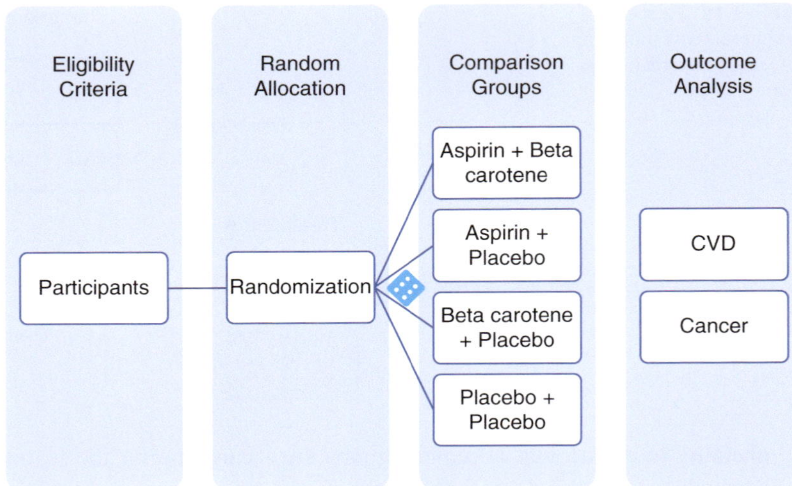

Fig. 3.20 Factorial trial design evaluating aspirin for cardiovascular disease (CVD) prevention and beta-carotene for cancer prevention

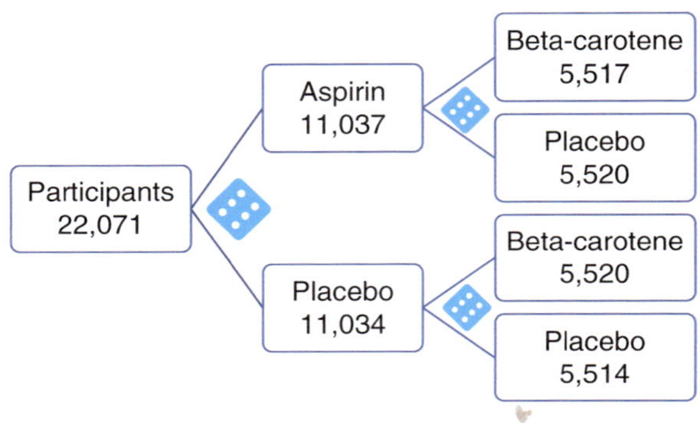

Fig. 3.21 Aspirin and beta-carotene used simultaneously in a factorial trial design

Table 3.19 Factorial design for examining the effects of aspirin and beta-carotene

		Aspirin +	Aspirin −
Beta carotene	+	Aspirin + Beta-carotene	Beta-carotene + Placebo
	−	Aspirin + Placebo	Placebo + Placebo

		Treatment A +	Treatment A −
Treatment B	+	Aspirin + Beta-carotene	Beta-carotene + Placebo
	−	Aspirin + Placebo	Placebo + Placebo

		Treatment A +	Treatment A −
Treatment B	+	Aspirin + Beta-carotene	Beta-carotene + Placebo
	−	Aspirin + Placebo	Placebo + Placebo

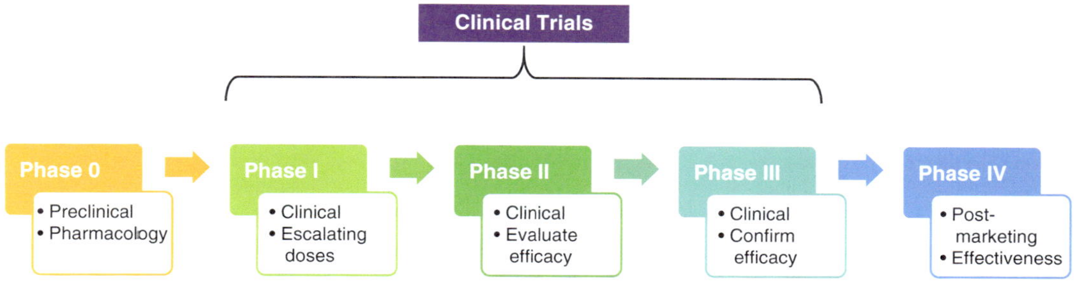

Fig. 3.22 Phases of a clinical trial

3.14 Phases of a Clinical Trial

Description
Clinical trials are research studies involving human volunteers to evaluate the safety and effectiveness of new medical interventions, such as drugs, vaccines, medical devices, or treatment combinations [1, 49]. They typically involve several phases as illustrated in Fig. 3.22.

Phase 0
Phase 0 trials, also known as exploratory or micro-dosing studies, are the earliest stage of clinical research, involving a very small number of participants, typically 10 to 15. There is generally no formal control group, and the primary goal is to gather preliminary data on a drug's pharmacokinetics (effects of the body on the drug, such as absorption, distribution, metabolism, and excretion) and pharmacodynamics (effects of the drug on the body). These trials use extremely low doses of the investigational drug, well below the therapeutic range, to minimize risk. They usually last for a short period, often just a few days.

Phase I
Phase I trials typically involve a small group of participants, usually between 20 and 100, and focus on assessing the safety and tolerability of a new drug. Participants are often healthy volunteers, although patients with the targeted condition may also be included. The drug is administered in increasing doses to determine the maximum tolerated dose (MTD), identify any side effects, and establish the appropriate dosage range. Typically, there is no formal control group in this phase.

Phase II
Phase II trials expand the sample size to a moderate range, typically involving 100 to 300 participants with the condition being treated. This phase aims to evaluate the drug's efficacy while continuing to monitor its safety. Participants are usually randomized into treatment groups, which may include a control group receiving a placebo or standard treatment for comparison. The primary objectives are to assess the drug's efficacy, evaluate the dose-response relationship, determine the optimal dose, and monitor safety and side effects.

Phase III
Phase III trials are large-scale studies that typically involve hundreds to thousands of participants, often ranging from 300 to over 3000. These trials are designed to confirm the efficacy and safety of the drug in a diverse population that resembles the general population with the condition. Participants are randomly assigned to treatment groups, including a control group receiving a placebo or standard care. The main objectives are to provide definitive evidence of the drug's efficacy, monitor adverse effects, and compare the new treatment against existing therapies. Successful completion of this phase is often required for regulatory approval and marketing of the drug.

Table 3.20 Comparison of clinical trial phases

Feature	Design	Population	Control group	Sample	Objective
Phase 0	Preclinical	Healthy volunteers	No	10–15	Bioavailability, pharmacodynamics[a], pharmacokinetics[b]
Phase I	Clinical	Healthy volunteers or patients	No	20–100	Escalating doses (MTD)[c], safety, short-term side effects
Phase II	Clinical	Patients	Yes	100–300	Evaluate efficacy, dose-response analysis, optimal dosing, short-term side effects
Phase III	Clinical	Patients	Yes	300–3000	Confirm efficacy, approval and license, short-term side effects
Phase IV	Post-marketing	Patient population	Yes/no	10,000–1000,000	Effectiveness in real-world use, rare or long-term side effects

[a]Pharmacodynamics: the effects of the drug on the body
[b]Pharmacokinetics: the effects of the body on the drug
[c]*MTD* maximum tolerated dose

Phase IV

Phase IV trials, also known as post-marketing surveillance studies, occur after a drug has received regulatory approval and is available for general use. The sample size for these studies can vary widely, often involving thousands of participants. The primary focus is to monitor the long-term effectiveness and safety of the drug in a broader patient population, including those with comorbidities and varying demographics. Many phase IV trials are observational in nature, where researchers observe and analyze data from patients who are already using the drug in routine clinical practice. These studies may or may not have a control group. Objectives of these trials include identifying rare or long-term side effects, such as carcinogenesis and teratogenesis, assessing the drug's performance in routine clinical practice, and gathering additional data to inform treatment guidelines and regulatory decisions. Findings from this phase can lead to label updates or, in rare cases, withdrawal of the drug from the market.

The characteristics of the different phases of clinical trials are summarized and compared in Table 3.20.

Conceptual Questions

1. Describe the different phases of clinical trials. What are the primary objectives and characteristics of each phase?
2. What is the purpose of phase 0 trials, and how do they differ from later phases? Discuss the significance of assessing pharmacokinetics and pharmacodynamics in this phase.
3. What are the objectives of phase I trials? What is meant by the "maximum tolerated dose," and why is this concept important during this phase?
4. What is meant by the "dose-response relationship," and why is this concept crucial in phase II trials?
5. What are the key objectives of phase II trials? How do these trials evaluate the efficacy of a treatment, and what role do short-term side effects play in this phase?
6. Discuss the significance of phase III trials in the clinical trial process. What is the importance of confirming efficacy and determining optimal dosing during this phase?
7. What occurs during phase IV trials, and why are they critical for post-marketing surveillance? Discuss the types of long-term effects that are evaluated in this phase.

Types of Literature Reviews

4

Contents

4.1 Reviews

A review is a comprehensive evaluation of existing research on a particular topic. It summarizes and interprets the findings of multiple studies to provide an overview of the present state of knowledge. Reviews can be categorized into several types based on their methodology, scope, and purpose, as illustrated in Fig. 4.1.

Narrative Review
A narrative review is a comprehensive *qualitative* synthesis of existing literature on a specific topic, typically authored by *experts* in the field. Its purpose is to provide a *broad* overview of present knowledge, trends, and gaps. Unlike systematic reviews, which adhere to a strict methodology for literature selection and appraisal, narrative reviews are generally less rigorous. They rely on the author's expertise and judgment in selecting and interpreting studies, which allows for greater flexibility but also increases the potential for bias [50, 51].

Narrative reviews aim to explain findings, consider different viewpoints, and highlight areas for future research. This makes them useful for suggesting new ideas or summarizing complicated topics for both general and expert audiences.

Example
A narrative review provided an overview of present best practices for bladder cancer, emphasizing the latest diagnostic and management strategies. It addressed challenges in pathology, including the evolving histological and molecular classifications of the disease, as well as advancements in personalized medicine and innovative imaging techniques. The review discusses the roles of radiotherapy and surgical management for both non-muscle-invasive and muscle-invasive bladder cancer while also highlighting the complexities involved in treating metastatic bladder cancer and the latest developments in systemic therapy. The review aimed to equip physicians with essential knowledge about contemporary issues and practices in the management of bladder cancer [52].

Rapid Review
A rapid review is a *time-limited* approach to synthesizing evidence, aimed at providing timely

J. Poorolajal, *Illustrated Epidemiology*, https://doi.org/10.1007/978-981-96-9566-9_4

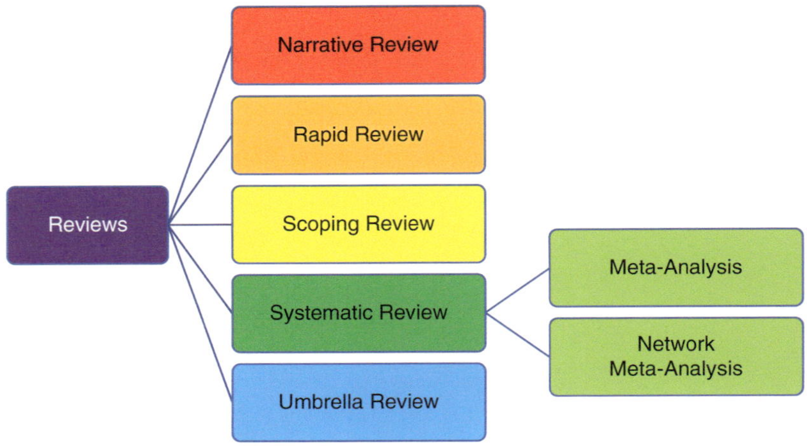

Fig. 4.1 Various types of reviews

and relevant information for decision-making, particularly in public health or policy contexts. It employs methods similar to those used in systematic reviews but simplifies or accelerates certain steps, such as narrowing the scope, utilizing fewer databases, or streamlining the appraisal process. While this expedites the review process, it may sacrifice some rigor for speed, potentially leading to reduced comprehensiveness and an increased risk of bias [53].

Rapid reviews are commonly utilized in policymaking, healthcare, and other fields where *timely* evidence is critical. They offer a practical balance between rigor and expediency, addressing urgent or emerging issues effectively.

Example
A rapid review investigated the psychological effects of quarantine during the coronavirus disease outbreak that began in December 2019, as many countries mandated isolation for individuals potentially exposed to the virus. The review analyzed 3166 papers and included 24 studies, most of which reported negative psychological outcomes such as post-traumatic stress symptoms, confusion, and anger. Identified stressors contributing to these effects included longer quarantine durations, fears of infection, frustration, boredom, inadequate supplies, insufficient information, financial loss, and stigma, with some studies suggesting potential long-lasting impacts. The review emphasized that when quarantine is necessary, it should be implemented for the shortest duration possible, accompanied by clear explanations of the rationale and protocols, as well as the provision of adequate supplies [54].

Scoping Review

A scoping review is a type of evidence synthesis that aims to map the *breadth* and *depth* of research on a specific topic or question. It identifies key concepts, types of evidence, and knowledge *gaps* within the literature. Unlike systematic reviews, which focus on a specific question and employ rigorous methodologies to assess the quality of included studies, scoping reviews are designed to provide an overview of existing literature. They aim to determine the extent and nature of available research, helping to identify knowledge gaps and inform future research directions [55].

Scoping reviews typically do not evaluate the quality of the included studies; instead, they focus on summarizing and categorizing findings to guide future research, policy development, or the planning of systematic reviews. They are particularly valuable for understanding the present state of research and framing new inquiries.

Example
A scoping review examined government policy measures aimed at addressing obesity among adults, emphasizing the global effectiveness of nutritional strategies implemented to reduce obesity prevalence. The review included 17 articles from seven countries (United States, United Kingdom, France, Mexico, Colombia, Chile, and

India), primarily consisting of observational, cross-sectional, and systematic reviews. The policies were categorized into three groups: food and beverage taxes ($n = 6$), food labeling ($n = 6$), and national campaigns ($n = 5$). While most policies resulted in only small changes in obesity metrics such as body mass index (BMI), two studies indicated that food labeling did not significantly impact weight status, whereas national campaigns demonstrated some success in reducing obesity risk. Notably, the sugar tax yielded more promising results, with evidence suggesting that higher tax rates correlated with greater declines in obesity prevalence. The findings aim to inform policymakers about effective food policies and encourage food industries to reformulate products to promote public health; however, the limited number of settings studied represents a key limitation, underscoring the need for further investigation into tax equity [56].

Systematic Review

A systematic review is a comprehensive research method that rigorously collects, analyzes, and synthesizes all existing evidence relevant to a specific question, aiming to minimize bias and provide reliable conclusions. It follows a predefined protocol that includes a thorough search of multiple databases, transparent inclusion and exclusion criteria, and a critical appraisal of study quality. The goal is to achieve objectivity and reproducibility while summarizing the findings of all pertinent studies [50, 51, 57].

Systematic reviews often incorporate meta-analyses to quantitatively summarize findings, although they can also be qualitative in nature. Widely regarded as the *gold standard* for evidence synthesis, systematic reviews are essential for informing clinical practice, policy decisions, and further research by providing a high level of evidence on a given topic.

Example

A systematic review was conducted to synthesize the existing literature on the association between birth weight and the risk of non-neurological childhood cancers. A comprehensive search of the PubMed, Web of Science, and Scopus databases was performed up to May 2023, resulting in the inclusion of 56 observational studies involving a total of 10,568,091 participants. The results indicated that low birth weight (<2500 g) was generally associated with a reduced risk for several types of childhood cancers, including acute lymphoblastic leukemia (OR: 0.82) and neuroblastoma (OR: 1.34). In contrast, high birth weight (>4000 g) was identified as a potential risk factor for various cancers, notably leukemia (OR: 1.30) and Wilms' tumor (OR: 1.49). These findings suggest that high birth weight may increase the risk of certain childhood cancers, while low birth weight may offer protective effects against some types [58].

Umbrella Review

An umbrella review is a comprehensive synthesis of systematic reviews and meta-analyses on a broad topic, providing a high-level overview of existing evidence. By systematically identifying, assessing, and combining evidence from these reviews, umbrella reviews offer a thorough overview of a research area, highlight knowledge gaps, and inform further research and decision-making. This type of review is particularly valuable in fields with a substantial volume of research or where systematic reviews address different aspects of a single topic. By consolidating the highest levels of evidence, umbrella reviews provide a clear, overarching perspective to guide decision-making, policy development, and future research priorities [59].

Example

An umbrella review aimed to identify, appraise, synthesize, and consolidate findings from published systematic reviews regarding the association between autoimmune diseases and adverse pregnancy outcomes. It included 33 systematic reviews encompassing 709 primary studies. The findings indicated that pregnant women with autoimmune conditions face a heightened risk of both maternal and fetal complications. Specific risks included increased miscarriage rates associated with Sjögren's syndrome (RR 8.85), systemic lupus erythematosus (SLE; OR 4.90), and thyroid autoimmunity (OR 2.77). Additionally, conditions such as type 1 diabetes and SLE were linked to higher risks of preeclampsia, while inflammatory bowel disease and thyroid autoimmunity increased the likelihood of gestational diabetes. The review also highlighted elevated risks for intrauterine growth restriction and delivering small-for-gestational-age babies among women with autoimmune disorders. Overall, the findings underscore the need for improved preconception to postnatal care for women with autoimmune conditions to mitigate these risks [60].

The characteristics of different types of reviews are compared in Table 4.1.

Conceptual Questions

1. How do the purposes of narrative reviews and systematic reviews differ, and what implications do these differences have for the interpretation of their findings?
2. Why is methodological rigor important in systematic reviews, and how does it contribute to the reliability of the conclusions drawn from the research?
3. In what situations would a rapid review be more appropriate than a systematic review? Discuss the trade-offs involved in choosing one method over the other.
4. How do scoping reviews contribute to identifying knowledge gaps in a research area, and what role do they play in shaping future research agendas?

4.2 Meta-Analysis

Description

Meta-analysis is a powerful statistical technique used in some systematic reviews. It combines data from multiple studies to provide a single, pooled estimate of the effect of an intervention or exposure. This combined estimate can offer a clearer picture of the evidence compared to examining individual studies in isolation [50, 51, 57, 61].

Example

In a systematic review and meta-analysis, researchers investigated the role of social support in preventing suicidal ideation. Figure 4.2 displays the forest plot summarizing the results of the meta-analysis [62].

Table 4.1 Comparison of review types

Types	Definition	Purpose	Rigor	Transparency	Methodology
Narrative review	A qualitative summary of existing literature	To provide a broad overview of present knowledge and trends	Low	Low	Subjective synthesis based on the author's expertise
Rapid review	A streamlined synthesis of evidence	To address urgent questions and provide timely information	Moderate	Moderate	Simplified synthesis with a focus on speed
Scoping review	A preliminary assessment of literature	To identify research gaps and map the existing evidence	Moderate	Moderate	Mapping of evidence to outline key concepts and gaps
Systematic review	A comprehensive synthesis of research evidence	To answer a specific research question with rigorous methods	High	High	Detailed methodology including meta-analysis (optional)
Umbrella review	A review of systematic reviews on a specific topic	To provide a comprehensive overview of existing systematic reviews and meta-analyses	High	High	Synthesis of syntheses, consolidating findings from multiple systematic reviews

Studies	log [Risk Ratio]	SE	Weight	Risk Ratio IV, Random, 95% CI
Arria et al. 2009	-0.18232	0.022197	57.4%	0.83 [0.80, 0.87]
Handley et al. 2012	-0.27444	0.138961	8.2%	0.76 [0.58, 1.00]
Kang et al. 2014	-0.13976	0.107966	12.6%	0.87 [0.70, 1.07]
Kim et al. 2014	-0.51879	0.154252	6.8%	0.60 [0.44, 0.81]
Wiebenga et al. 2021	-0.15082	0.097375	14.9%	0.86 [0.71, 1.04]
Total (95% CI)			**100.0%**	**0.82 [0.75, 0.89]**

Heterogeneity: $Tau^2 = 0.00$; $Chi^2 = 5.40$, df = 4 (P = 0.25); $I^2 = 26\%$
Test for overall effect: Z = 4.77 (P < 0.00001)

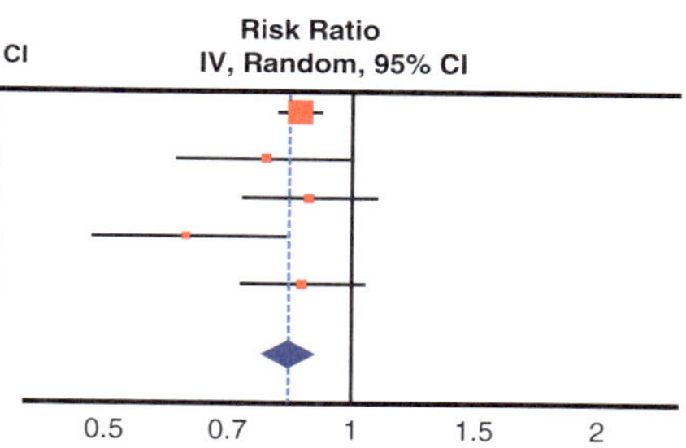

Fig. 4.2 A typical forest plot illustrating the results of a meta-analysis

- Squares: Represent point estimates, indicating the average effect size observed in each study.
- Larger square area: Represents a larger study sample size.
- Horizontal lines: Indicate confidence intervals, reflecting the range within which the true effect size is likely to fall.
- Solid vertical line: Indicates no effect.
- Dashed vertical line: Represents the average effect size across all included studies.
- Vertical diameter of the diamond shape: Represents the summary measure of the effect size.
- Horizontal diameter of the diamond shape: Indicates the confidence interval of the summary measure.
- Heterogeneity Statistics: $Tau^2 = 0.00$ (no substantial between-study variance).
- $Chi^2 = 5.40$, df = 4, P = 0.25 (no significant heterogeneity).
- $I^2 = 26\%$ (low heterogeneity).
- Test for Overall Effect: Z = 4.77, P 0.00001 (highly statistically significant pooled result).

Confidence intervals that cross the solid vertical line signify a non-statistically significant difference between the intervention and control groups.

Conceptual Questions

1. How does meta-analysis improve the reliability of findings compared to individual studies?
2. What are the implications of using pooled estimates in understanding the effect of an intervention?
3. In what ways can the visualization of data through forest plots aid in interpreting the results of a meta-analysis?
4. How do confidence intervals in a meta-analysis inform researchers about the precision of effect size estimates?
5. What does it mean when confidence intervals cross the solid vertical line in a forest plot, and how should this influence the interpretation of results?
6. How can the size of the squares in a forest plot reflect the significance of study findings in a meta-analysis?
7. What role does the assessment of study heterogeneity play in the validity of a meta-analysis?
8. How does the summary measure of effect size contribute to the overall conclusions drawn from a meta-analysis?

4.3 Network Meta-Analysis

Description

Network meta-analysis (NMA) is a powerful statistical technique that goes beyond traditional pairwise comparisons. It enables researchers to compare multiple interventions (treatments, therapies) simultaneously in a single analysis by combining both direct and indirect evidences from a network of studies. Direct evidence includes studies that directly compare two interventions (such as treatment A vs. treatment B), while indirect evidence includes studies that do not directly compare the interventions of interest but share a common comparator (e.g., both studies compare treatment A vs. placebo and treatment B vs. placebo). By analyzing these comparisons together, NMA can estimate the effectiveness of treatment A compared to treatment B even when there is no direct study testing them [51, 63].

Example 1
Consider a hypothetical network meta-analysis in which researchers are investigating the most effective medication for lowering blood pressure, as illustrated in Fig. 4.3. Several medications are available, but not all have been directly compared in clinical trials.

The medications under investigation include:

- Medication A: Beta-blocker.
- Medication B: Thiazide diuretic.
- Medication C: Angiotensin-converting enzyme (ACE) inhibitor.
- Medication D: Angiotensin II receptor blocker (ARB).
- Medication E: Calcium channel blocker (CCB), dihydropyridine type.
- Medication F: Placebo (control).

Traditional pairwise meta-analysis can only compare medications individually, such as medication A vs. placebo, medication B vs. placebo, and so on. This approach does not provide insights into how medication A compares to medication E if they have not been directly compared head-to-head.

To overcome this limitation, researchers utilize a network diagram to illustrate which medications have been directly compared in trials. Figure 4.3 displays a typical network diagram summarizing the results of the hypothetical NMA:

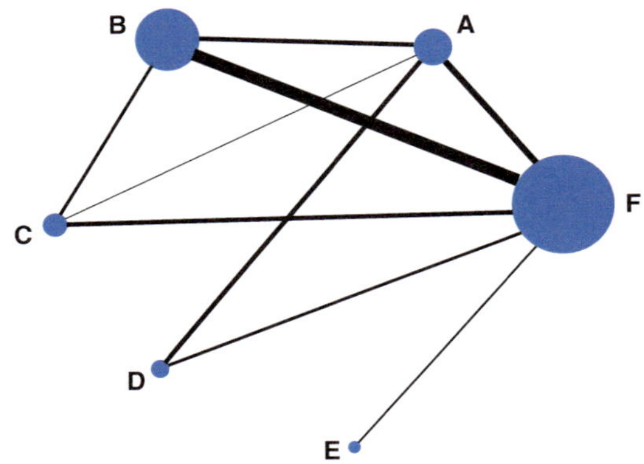

Fig. 4.3 A typical network diagram illustrating the results of a network meta-analysis

- Nodes: Each node represents a different treatment.
- Larger nodes: The size of each node indicates the number of participants involved in studies for that treatment.
- Edges (lines): The lines connecting the nodes signify direct comparisons between treatments.
- Thicker lines: The thickness of the lines indicates the number of trials that have directly compared the two treatments.

For NMA to be valid, ideally all trials in the network should be similar in terms of factors that could influence treatment effects, known as treatment effect modifiers. This assumption can be broken down into three key aspects: homogeneity, transitivity, and consistency.

Homogeneity
Description: Homogeneity refers to the assumption that the treatment effects across studies included in the NMA are similar. This means that the variation in treatment effects is not due to differences in study populations, interventions, or outcomes.

Example: If you are comparing the effectiveness of three different pain relief medications (A, B, and C) in various studies, homogeneity assumes that the effect of medication A compared to B is consistent across all studies included in the analysis.

Violation Implications: If homogeneity is violated, it could indicate that the studies are too heterogeneous (i.e., they differ significantly in design, population, or context), leading to unreliable pooled estimates. This can result in misleading conclusions about the effectiveness of treatments.

Transitivity

Description: Transitivity is the assumption that the studies included in the NMA are comparable in terms of their populations, interventions, and outcomes, allowing for indirect comparisons. This means that if treatment A is compared to B and B to C, then we can infer a comparison between A and C.

Example: Suppose you have studies comparing medication A to B and medication B to C. Transitivity assumes that the populations and conditions in these studies are sufficiently similar, allowing you to infer the effectiveness of A compared to C based on the other comparisons.

Violation Implications: If transitivity is violated, it may lead to incorrect conclusions about the relative effectiveness of treatments because the groups being compared may not be comparable. This can result in biased estimates and undermine the validity of the indirect comparisons.

Consistency

Description: Consistency refers to the agreement between direct and indirect evidence regarding treatment effects. In other words, the treatment effect estimated from direct comparisons should align with the treatment effect inferred from indirect comparisons.

Example: If direct comparisons show that medication A is more effective than medication B, and the indirect comparison (through medication C) also suggests that A is more effective than B, then consistency holds.

Violation Implications: If consistency is violated, it indicates a discrepancy between direct and indirect evidence, which can lead to conflicting conclusions about the effectiveness of treatments. This can arise from biases in the studies or differences in the populations studied, leading to uncertainty in the overall conclusions of the NMA.

The three fundamental assumptions of homogeneity, transitivity, and consistency in network meta-analysis (NMA) can be illustrated through a hypothetical example comparing the effects of three antidepressants—sertraline, fluoxetine, and citalopram—in the treatment of depression:

- *Homogeneity*: Homogeneity implies that results across different studies regarding the effectiveness of the three antidepressants are consistent. For example, if one study concludes that sertraline is the most effective and citalopram the least effective, all studies should yield similar conclusions. However, if some studies report fluoxetine as either more effective or less effective than the other two drugs, the assumption of homogeneity is violated, indicating heterogeneity and reducing the reliability of the findings.
- *Transitivity*: Transitivity requires that all treatments are compared under similar conditions, including patient characteristics, outcome measures, prescribed doses, and follow-up duration. For example, the transitivity assumption holds if all three drugs are prescribed for moderate depression at specific doses (e.g., sertraline 100 mg, fluoxetine 50 mg, and citalopram 40 mg) and symptoms are assessed after 4 weeks using a clinician-rated scale. However, this assumption is violated if comparisons involve patients with varying depression severity (e.g., mild, moderate, or severe), different doses, diverse outcome measures (e.g., clinician-rated vs. self-reported), or inconsistent follow-up durations (e.g., 4 weeks vs. 6 weeks). Such violations compromise the validity of the comparisons.
- *Consistency*: Consistency refers to agreement between results obtained from direct comparisons and those derived from indirect comparisons. For example, if a direct comparison shows that sertraline is more effective than fluoxetine, the indirect comparison (e.g., through citalopram) should support the same conclusion. If the indirect comparison contradicts the direct findings, the consistency assumption is violated, suggesting potential biases or methodological issues in the analysis.

Example 2

A network meta-analysis (NMA) aimed to compare various pharmaceutical therapies for treating obesity to identify the most effective treatment options for patients and physicians. The analysis included 96 randomized controlled trials, comprising 68 with both men and women, 23 with women only, and five with men only. The results indicated that the best-ranked treatments for both men and women were semaglutide, 2.4 mg, followed by hydroxycitric acid combined with supervised walking and a 2000-kcal diet, phentermine hydrochloride with behavioral therapy, and liraglutide with dietary advice. Overall, the findings suggest that semaglutide is a highly effective treatment for obesity in both sexes [64].

Conceptual Questions

1. What distinguishes network meta-analysis (NMA) from traditional pairwise meta-analysis? Discuss the advantages of using NMA in clinical research.
2. Explain the difference between direct evidence and indirect evidence in the context of NMA. How does the combination of both types of evidence enhance the analysis?
3. How can researchers interpret a network diagram? What do the size of the nodes and the thickness of the connecting lines indicate about the studies included in the analysis?
4. What is homogeneity in the context of NMA, and why is it important for trials included in the analysis to be similar in terms of patient characteristics, interventions, and outcomes?
5. What is transitivity in NMA, and how does it relate to the comparability of treatment conditions across trials? Why is this assumption critical for valid indirect comparisons?
6. What is consistency in NMA, and how can researchers assess whether direct and indirect evidences are in agreement? What are the implications if consistency is violated?

Sampling Methods in Epidemiology

5

Contents

5.1 Populations in Epidemiological Research

Epidemiologists use a variety of terms to describe groups of people, and these terms are often used inconsistently. Below are some common terms used in epidemiological research to describe populations:

Target Population
Definition: The entire group of individuals to whom the researcher wants to generalize the study findings [1]. It is a broader population from which the study sample is drawn, as shown in Fig. 5.1.

Example: All adults aged 18–65 living in a country with type 2 diabetes

Source Population
Definition: The source population, also known as the sampling frame, is the population from which the study population is actually drawn [1]. It is often a practical representation of the target population that is available for study, often due to geographical, temporal, or logistical limitations, as illustrated in Fig. 5.1.

Example: All adults aged 18–65 with type 2 diabetes enrolled in a specific healthcare system or living in a particular city in the country

Study Population (Sample)
Definition: The group of individuals who actually participate in the study [1]. It is a subset of the source population, as shown in Fig. 5.1.

J. Poorolajal, *Illustrated Epidemiology*, https://doi.org/10.1007/978-981-96-9566-9_5

Example: A random sample of 1000 adults aged 18–65 with type 2 diabetes living in a specific city in the country

Reference Population

Definition: The standard group against which a studied population is compared [1]. This group can either be the general population or a specific subset that does not have the exposure or outcome of interest.

Example: Adults without type 2 diabetes matched for age, sex, and other relevant factors as the reference group for a case-control study

Synonymy

Source population; Base population; Sampling frame

Study population; Study sample; Study group

Conceptual Questions

1. What are the key differences between the target population, source population, study population, and reference population in epidemiological research? Provide definitions and examples for each.
2. Why is it important for researchers to clearly define the target population in their studies? How does the choice of target population affect the generalizability of the study findings?
3. Discuss the significance of the source population (sampling frame) in the context of epidemiological studies. What challenges might researchers face when selecting a source population?
4. What role does the reference population play in comparative studies, such as case-control studies? How can the selection of a reference population impact the interpretation of study results?
5. Provide an example of how the differences between the target population and the source population could lead to challenges in interpreting the results of an epidemiological study.

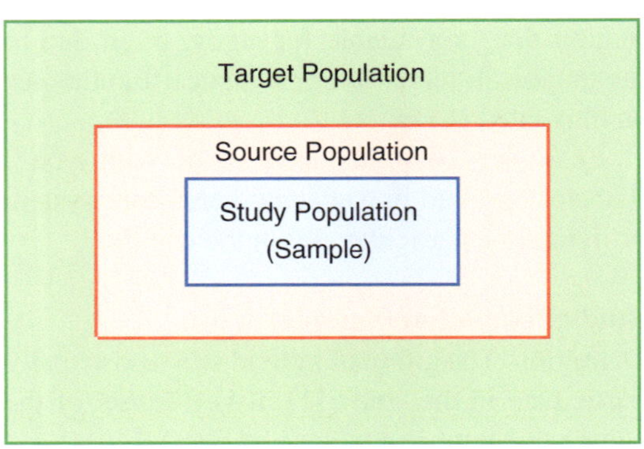

Fig. 5.1 Population types in epidemiology

5.2 Random Sampling Versus Random Allocation

Random sampling and random allocation are often confused, but they serve different purposes in research. Table 5.1 illustrates this distinction.

Random Sampling

Random sampling is the process of selecting a *representative* subset of individuals from a larger population (the entire group of interest). This method ensures that every individual in the population has an equal chance of being chosen, thereby minimizing selection bias and enhancing *generalizability*, as illustrated in Fig. 5.2 [1, 4].

Example

Researchers aimed to assess the prevalence of psychiatric distress among college students at Hamadan University of Medical Sciences. To achieve this, a random sample of 1259 students was selected from the whole university students. This sampling method ensured that the study participants accurately represented the diverse

Table 5.1 Key differences between random sampling and random allocation

Feature	Random sampling	Random allocation
Types of study	Observational studies	Interventional studies
Purpose	Increase external validity	Increase internal validity
Ensures	Generalizability	Comparability

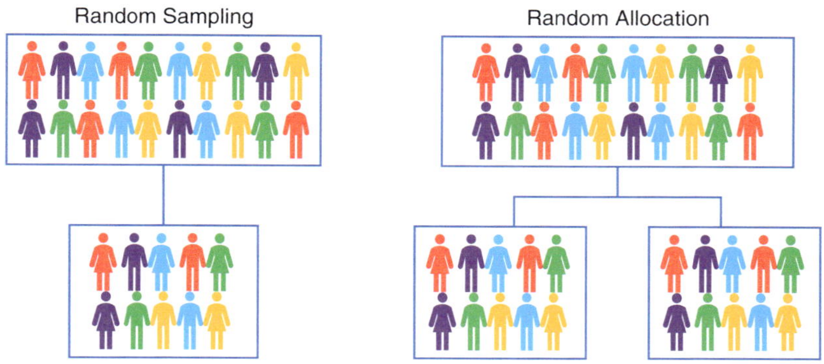

Fig. 5.2 Random sampling vs. random allocation

demographics of the university student body, including factors such as age, gender, and academic level [65].

Random Allocation
Random allocation is the process of randomly assigning participants from a sample to different groups within an experiment. This is done in order to compare the effects of something, such as a new medication [2, 4]. Figure 5.2 illustrates this process.

Example
Researchers conducted a randomized controlled trial to evaluate the effects of tranexamic acid and phenylephrine on bleeding during endoscopic sinus surgery. Sixty eligible patients were randomly assigned to receive either a combination of phenylephrine and tranexamic acid ($n = 30$) or phenylephrine alone ($n = 30$). This random allocation minimizes bias and ensures *comparability* between the groups at the start of the study [66].

Conceptual Questions
1. What are the key differences between random sampling and random allocation? Provide definitions and examples for each to illustrate their distinct purposes in research.
2. Why is random sampling important for observational studies? How does it contribute to the external validity of the research findings?
3. Discuss how random allocation enhances internal validity in interventional studies. Why is internal validity crucial for the reliability of experimental results?
4. Explain how random allocation minimizes bias in clinical trials. What types of biases can it help to prevent, and why is this important for the integrity of the study?
5. How does the size of the sample impact the effectiveness of random sampling and random allocation? What considerations should researchers keep in mind regarding sample size?

5.3 Sampling Methods

Sampling methods can be broadly categorized into probability sampling (random sampling) and non-probability sampling. Non-probability sampling, such as convenience sampling, is a method of selecting individuals from a population where not all members have an equal chance of being chosen. This approach can introduce bias and limit the generalizability of the results. In contrast, probability sampling ensures that every individual in the population has an *equal* chance of being selected. This is achieved through various methods, including systematic random sampling, simple random sampling, stratified random sampling, and cluster random sampling, as illustrated in Fig. 5.3.

Conceptual Questions
1. What are the key differences between probability sampling and non-probability sampling? Provide examples of each.
2. How does non-probability sampling, such as convenience sampling, affect the potential for

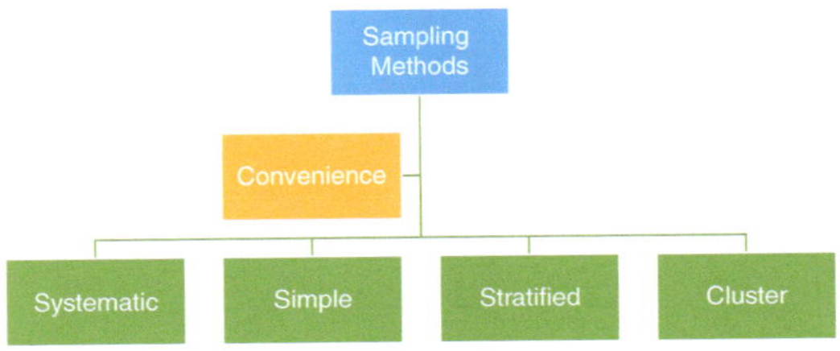

Fig. 5.3 Various approaches to sampling methods

bias in research findings? In what ways can this impact the generalizability of the results?
3. In what scenarios might a researcher choose non-probability sampling over probability sampling? Discuss the advantages and disadvantages of this choice.
4. Describe the various methods of probability sampling. How does each method ensure that every individual has an equal chance of being selected?

5.4 Convenience Sampling

Description

Convenience sampling is a non-probability sampling method where participants are chosen for a study based on their *availability* and *accessibility* to the researcher, as illustrated in Fig. 5.4. This means that the researcher selects individuals who are convenient at the time, rather than using a random selection process [67].

Advantages

1. Ease of access: Researchers can quickly and easily access participants, as they select individuals who are readily available, such as friends, colleagues, or people in a specific location.
2. Cost-effective: Convenience sampling often requires fewer resources in terms of time, money, and effort compared to more complex sampling methods.
3. Speed: Data collection can be completed more rapidly, making it suitable for exploratory research or studies with tight deadlines.
4. Useful for preliminary research: It can provide initial insights and generate hypotheses for further investigation, especially in qualitative studies.

Disadvantages

1. Bias: The sample may not be representative of the broader population, leading to selection bias. This can skew results and limit the validity of conclusions.
2. Limited generalizability: Findings from convenience samples may not be applicable to the entire population, as they may reflect the characteristics of only a specific subgroup.

Example 1

Imagine municipal officials planning to evaluate public attitudes and opinions about city services by conducting a survey using a multiple-choice questionnaire. To achieve this, they will target individuals in high-traffic areas such as malls, metro stations, cafeterias, streets, and other crowded locations.

Example 2

A study aimed to assess childhood obesity levels in local populations by utilizing convenience sampling of children presenting to hospital-based outpatient clinics. Recognizing childhood obesity as a critical public health issue linked to various pediatric comorbidities, the researchers hypothesized that samples from clinic visits could yield representative local estimates of obesity from 2007 to 2013, potentially offering more accurate, timely, and cost-effective data compared to national surveys. However, the results indicated that the hospital-based sample did not effectively serve as a surrogate for the broader population [68].

Conceptual Questions

1. What is convenience sampling, and how does it differ from probability sampling methods? Discuss the key characteristics that define convenience sampling.
2. What are the main limitations of convenience sampling? How can these limitations impact the validity and reliability of research findings?

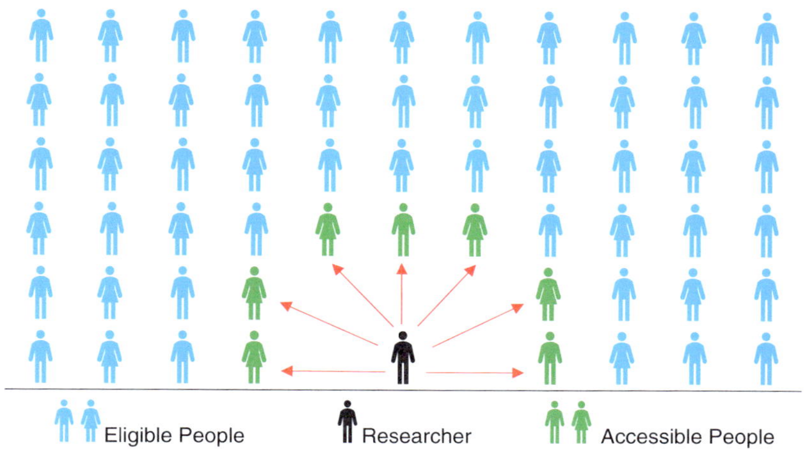

Fig. 5.4 Convenience sampling process

3. How does the use of convenience sampling affect the generalizability of study results to the broader population? Provide examples to illustrate your points.
4. Provide examples of research scenarios where convenience sampling might be an appropriate choice. What factors would lead researchers to select this method over more rigorous sampling techniques?

5.5 Systematic Random Sampling

Description

Systematic random sampling is a *probability* sampling method that begins with a random "starting point" and then selects every "*k*th" element from a population list. The sampling interval "*k*" is calculated by dividing the total population size "*N*" by the desired sample size "*n*" [67].

As illustrated in Fig. 5.5, to create a random sample of six people from a population of 18 individuals, we first determine the sampling interval (k). This is calculated as:

$$k = \frac{N}{n} = \frac{18}{6} = 3$$

Next, we randomly select a starting point from the first three individuals. This could be done using a random number generator or other method. Once we have the starting point, we systematically select every third individual from the list until we have six people in our sample.

Advantages

1. Simplicity: The method is straightforward to implement. Once a random starting point is chosen, researchers can easily select subsequent participants at regular intervals.
2. Reduced bias: Systematic random sampling helps minimize selection bias compared to convenience sampling, as it involves a random starting point and a fixed interval for selection.
3. Efficient data collection: This method can be more efficient than simple random sampling, especially when dealing with large populations, as it reduces the time and effort needed to select participants.

Disadvantages

1. Risk of periodicity: If there is a hidden pattern or periodicity in the population list (e.g., every tenth person has similar characteristics), it can lead to biased samples that do not accurately represent the population.
2. Dependence on population order: The effectiveness of systematic sampling relies on how the population is organized. If the list is not random or is sorted in a way that relates to the study variable, the sample may be unrepresentative.

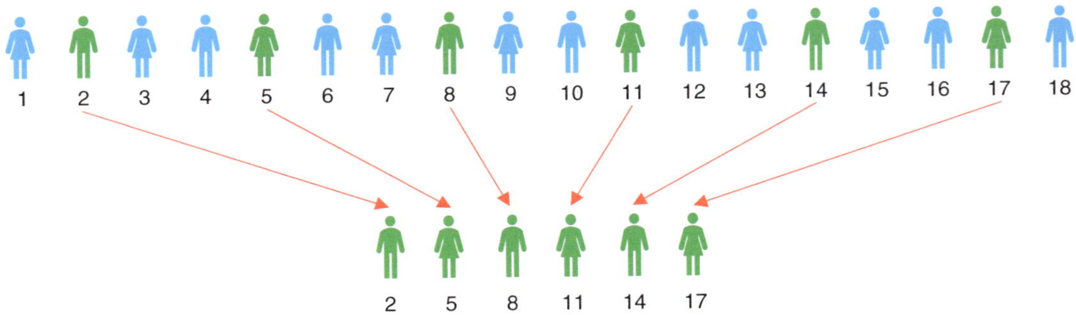

Fig. 5.5 Systematic random sampling process

Example 1
Let's consider a hypothetical company with 1000 employees looking to assess employee satisfaction. To achieve this, they can select a random sample of 50 employees. This can be done through systematic random sampling. In this method, they would first determine the sampling interval (k) by dividing the total number of employees (1000) by the desired sample size (50). This calculation gives them a sampling interval of 20 ($k = 1000/50 = 20$).

Next, they would randomly select a number between 1 and 20 as the "starting point" on their employee list. For example, if the chosen starting point is 6, they would then survey every 20th employee on the list starting from employee number 6 (26th, 46th, 66th, 86th, etc.). This process continues until they reach a sample size of 50 employees.

Example 2
A study employed a systematic random sampling method to investigate the epidemiology, clinical characteristics, and associated costs of acute poisoning in the emergency department of the largest tertiary care healthcare center. The researchers conducted a retrospective review of health records for patients admitted due to poisoning in Qatar between January 2015 and December 2019. They initiated the sampling by randomly selecting the seventh patient as a starting point and then included every tenth patient thereafter (17th, 27th, 37th, etc.). Ultimately, a total of 401 cases were obtained from 4006 electronic medical records using this systematic random sampling technique. This method is particularly efficient for larger samples, as it provides a representative subset of the population, ensuring that the data collected reflects broader trends in acute poisoning cases [69].

Conceptual Questions
1. What is systematic random sampling, and how does it differ from simple random sampling? Describe the step-by-step process involved in systematic random sampling.
2. Explain how the sampling interval (k) is calculated in systematic random sampling. Why is this calculation important for the sampling process?
3. Why is the selection of a random starting point crucial in systematic random sampling? What methods can be used to ensure that this starting point is truly random?
4. What are the advantages of using systematic random sampling compared to other sampling methods? In what scenarios might this method be particularly beneficial?

5.6 Simple Random Sampling

Description
Simple random sampling is a type of *probability* sampling in which a subset of individuals is randomly selected from a population. In this method, each member of the population has an *equal* probability of being chosen [1, 67]. This approach ensures that the randomly selected sample is a *miniature* representation of the entire population, as illustrated in Fig. 5.6.

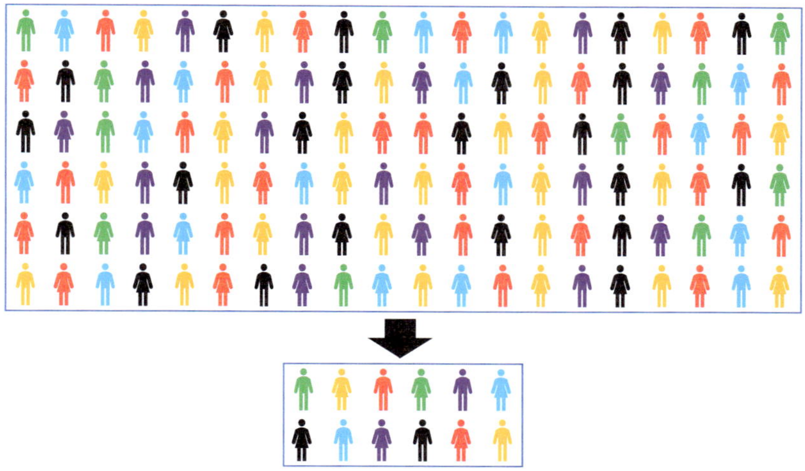

Fig. 5.6 Simple random sampling process

Advantages

1. Equal probability: Every member of the population has an equal chance of being selected, which helps eliminate selection bias and enhances the representativeness of the sample.
2. Statistical validity: Simple random sampling allows for the use of various statistical techniques and formulas, facilitating the calculation of confidence intervals and margins of error.
3. Generalizability: Results obtained from a simple random sample can often be generalized to the larger population, assuming the sample is adequately sized.

Disadvantages

1. Practicality: It can be difficult to obtain a complete list of the population, especially in large or dispersed populations, making it challenging to implement.
2. Cost and time: Depending on the population size, simple random sampling may require significant time and resources to ensure that every member has an equal chance of selection.
3. Sampling error: While simple random sampling reduces bias, it does not eliminate sampling error. A small sample may still not accurately reflect the population, especially if the sample size is inadequate.

Example 1

As a hypothetical example, imagine a school with 500 students where the administration aims to survey 100 of them about their after-school activity preferences using simple random sampling. Each student is assigned a unique number from 1 to 500, and a random number generator is used to select 100 unique numbers, ensuring that every student has an equal chance of being chosen. The selected students are then contacted to complete a survey that includes questions about their present activities and interests in new ones.

Example 2

A study employed simple random sampling to examine the association between psychiatric disorders and risky behaviors among Iranian university students. Conducted in 2017, the national survey included 4261 students from 13 medical science universities across the country. This sampling method ensured that each student had an equal chance of being selected, which helped to create a representative sample of the broader student population. The survey assessed various health-risk behaviors, including cigarette smoking, illicit drug use, alcohol consumption, unprotected sexual intercourse, suicidal ideation, suicide attempts, and Internet addiction. The findings indicated that 39% of the students had some level of psychiatric disorder, and 37.3% engaged in at least one risky behavior. The use of simple random sampling facilitated a robust analysis of the prevalence of psychiatric disorders and their relationship with risky behaviors in this demographic [70].

Conceptual Questions

1. What is simple random sampling, and how does it ensure that each member of the population has an equal chance of being selected? Discuss the key characteristics that define this sampling method.
2. Describe the step-by-step process of conducting simple random sampling, using the school example provided. What tools or methods can be used to select the sample?
3. What are the advantages of using simple random sampling in research? How does it contribute to the validity and reliability of study findings?
4. What are some potential limitations or challenges associated with simple random sampling? How might these challenges affect the results of a study?

5.7 Stratified Random Sampling

Description

Stratified random sampling is a *probability* sampling method that involves dividing a population into smaller, *homogeneous* groups known as *strata* based on specific characteristics (e.g., age, gender, and income). Random samples are then taken from each stratum to create a sample that accurately reflects the population's diversity, as shown in Fig. 5.7 [1, 67].

This method is particularly useful when dealing with *heterogeneous* populations where a simple random sample might not adequately represent all subgroups. By stratifying the population, researchers can ensure that their sample reflects the composition of the population and minimize sampling bias.

There are two primary types of stratified random sampling:

Proportionate Stratified Sampling

This method maintains the same proportions of each stratum in the sample as in the population. For instance, if a population is 60% female and 40% male, a proportionate sample would also be 60% female and 40% male.

Disproportionate Stratified Sampling

This method involves deliberately oversampling or undersampling specific strata to increase their representation in the sample. This method is useful when certain subgroups are of particular interest and need more representation in the sample. For example, in a population with 70%

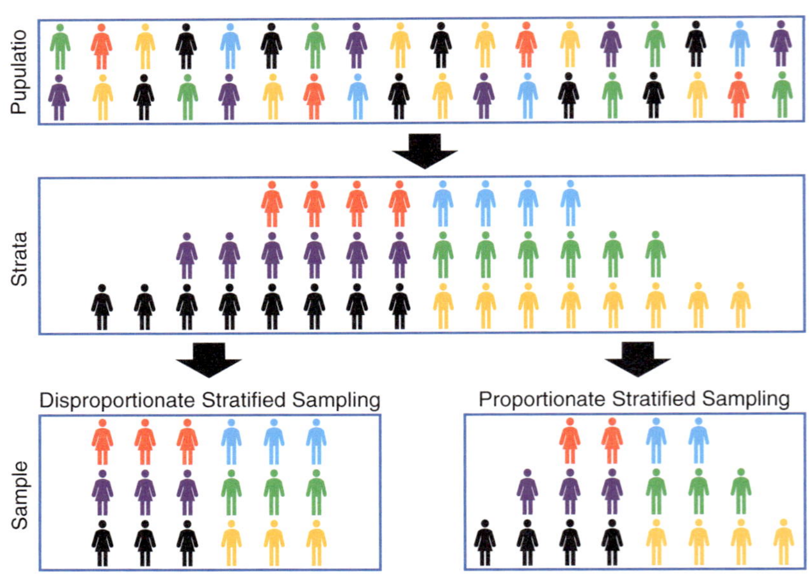

Fig. 5.7 Stratified random sampling process

young adults and 30% seniors, a disproportionate stratified sample might have 50% young adults and 50% seniors.

Advantages

1. Increased precision: By dividing the population into distinct subgroups (strata) and sampling from each, stratified random sampling often yields more precise estimates than simple random sampling, especially when there are significant differences between strata.
2. Enhanced representativeness: This method ensures that all relevant subgroups are represented in the sample, which can improve the generalizability of the results to the entire population.
3. Targeted analysis: Researchers can analyze specific subgroups more effectively, allowing for insights into the differences and similarities among strata.

Disadvantages

1. Complexity: The process of identifying and defining strata can be complex and time-consuming, requiring detailed knowledge of the population.
2. Need for complete population information: Effective stratified sampling requires a complete list of the population and information about the characteristics used to define the strata, which may not always be available.
3. Potential for misclassification: If individuals are incorrectly assigned to strata, it can lead to biased results and affect the overall validity of the findings.
4. Increased costs: Stratified random sampling can be more resource-intensive than simple random sampling due to the additional steps involved in stratification and the need to sample from multiple groups.

Example

Researchers are investigating COVID-19 vaccination rates among adults in a hypothetical city, as illustrated in Fig. 5.8. To anticipate variations in vaccination rates based on age and socioeconomic status, they have stratified the population into two groups:

- Socioeconomic status: low, middle, and high income
- Age: 18–40, 41–64, and 65+ years

To achieve a sample size of 900 individuals, researchers plan to randomly select 100 adults from each of the nine age-income strata combinations (3 income levels × 3 age groups × 100 individuals). For example, 100 individuals aged 18–40 with low income will be randomly selected, and this process will be repeated for all other strata. Random digit dialing within zip codes associated with each socioeconomic status will be used for sample selection.

Conceptual Questions

1. What is stratified random sampling, and why is it particularly useful for heterogeneous populations? Discuss how this method helps to minimize sampling bias.
2. How do researchers determine the strata when conducting stratified random sampling? What characteristics might be used to create these groups, and why are they important?
3. Explain the differences between proportionate stratified sampling and disproportionate

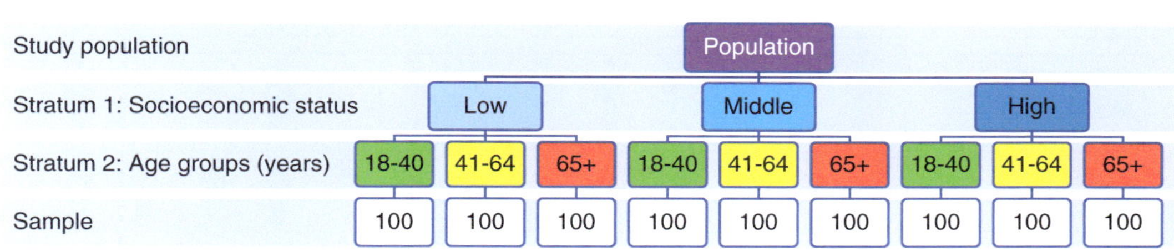

Fig. 5.8 Disproportionate stratified random sample by socioeconomic status and age

stratified sampling. In what situations would a researcher choose one method over the other?

4. Describe the process of selecting samples from each stratum in stratified random sampling. How does this process ensure that the sample reflects the diversity of the population?
5. What are the advantages of using stratified random sampling compared to simple random sampling? How does it improve the representativeness of the sample?

5.8 Cluster Random Sampling

Description

Cluster random sampling is a *probability* sampling method that involves dividing a population into geographically defined groups (clusters), such as neighborhoods or schools. Researchers then randomly select *some* of these clusters to form a sample. This method is often used to study large populations spread across a wide geographical area or when natural groupings exist within the population based on factors like race, ethnicity, or socioeconomic status [67].

Example 1

Researchers aim to study the prevalence of hypertension in a rural area with seven villages, as illustrated in Fig. 5.9. For this study, each village is considered a cluster. Three villages are randomly selected from the seven for inclusion in the study. All adult residents, both male and female, aged 18–65 within the chosen villages will participate in the research.

Advantages

1. Cost-effective: Cluster random sampling can significantly reduce costs associated with data collection, especially in large populations spread over wide geographic areas, by allowing researchers to focus on specific clusters rather than the entire population.
2. Efficiency: It simplifies the logistics of data collection, making it easier to manage and coordinate efforts, as researchers can gather data from multiple individuals within a single location.
3. Time-saving: Researchers can collect data more quickly by sampling entire clusters rather than individuals scattered across a large area.

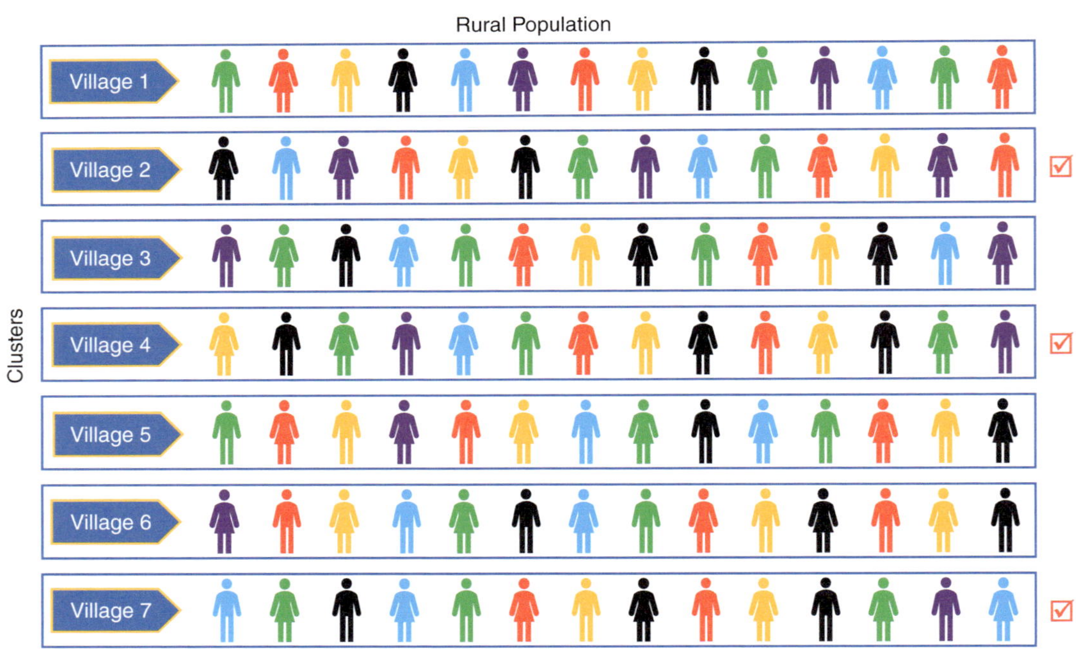

Fig. 5.9 Cluster random sampling process

Disadvantages

1. Potential for bias: If the selected clusters are not representative of the overall population, the results may be biased, affecting the validity of the findings.
2. Complex analysis: Analyzing data from cluster samples can be more complicated, requiring specialized statistical techniques to account for the cluster design and its potential effects on the results.
3. Higher sample size needed: Cluster sampling typically requires a larger sample size to achieve the same level of precision as other sampling methods.

Example 2

In a study investigating the factors influencing bone mass abnormalities among postmenopausal women in Tibet, China, a multistage cluster sampling technique was employed to randomly select a total of 229 participants from six counties, as illustrated in Fig. 5.10. The sampling process consisted of several stages:

- *Stage 1*: Three out of six regions were randomly selected (cluster level 1, gray rectangles).
- *Stage 2*: One to three counties were randomly chosen from each selected region (cluster level 2, orange rectangles), resulting in a total of six counties.
- *Stage 3*: Two townships were randomly selected from each county (cluster level 3, green rectangles).
- *Stage 4*: Two to three urban residential or rural village communities were randomly chosen from each township (cluster level 4, blue rectangles).
- *Stage 5*: All residents aged over 15 years in the selected communities were included in the study.

This systematic approach ensured a representative sample of the population. The analysis revealed that the prevalence of osteopenia and osteoporosis among the participants was 54.6% and 9.6%, respectively, highlighting significant public health concerns within this demographic [71].

Conceptual Questions

1. What is cluster random sampling, and how does it differ from other probability sampling methods such as simple random sampling and stratified random sampling? Discuss the key characteristics that define this method.
2. Why might researchers choose cluster random sampling when studying large populations? What are the advantages of using clusters, especially in geographically dispersed populations?
3. Describe the process of selecting clusters in cluster random sampling. How do researchers ensure that the selection of clusters is random, and what tools or methods might they use?
4. What are the advantages of using cluster random sampling compared to other sampling methods? How does this method help reduce

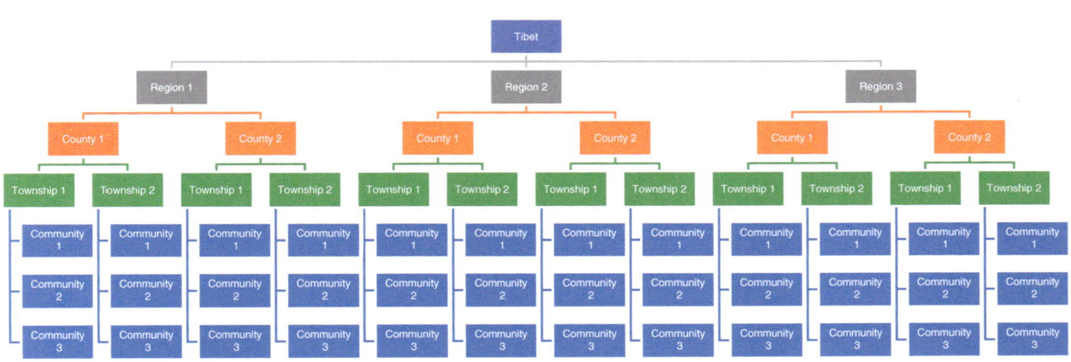

Fig. 5.10 Multistage cluster sampling technique for randomly selecting 229 participants

costs and logistical challenges in data collection?
5. How does cluster sampling reduce costs compared to other sampling methods, and in what scenarios is this particularly beneficial?
6. Why might cluster sampling lead to higher sampling error compared to simple random sampling or stratified sampling?

5.9 Stratified Random Sampling Versus Cluster Random Sampling

Both stratified and cluster sampling are probability sampling methods, but they differ in how the population is divided and sampled. Table 5.2 summarizes the differences between them.

In *stratified* random sampling, the population is divided into homogeneous subgroups (strata) based on specific characteristics such as age, gender, or income. A random sample is then selected from *each stratum*. This method aims to ensure the representation of different subgroups within the population and can improve the precision of estimates.

In *cluster* random sampling, the population is divided into heterogeneous groups, often based on geographical location or naturally occurring groupings such as schools or neighborhoods. Data is then collected from all individuals within the *randomly selected clusters*. This method is generally more efficient and cost-effective for large, geographically dispersed populations.

As illustrated in Fig. 5.11, the processes can be summarized as follows:

Table 5.2 Comparison of stratified random sampling and cluster random sampling

Characteristics	Stratified random sampling	Cluster random sampling
Goal	Enhance precision	Reduce costs
Selection	Random selection from all defined strata	Random selection from a few preselected clusters
Division	Researcher-defined groups (strata)	Naturally occurring groups (clusters)
Internal homogeneity	Homogeneous within each stratum	Heterogeneous within each cluster
External homogeneity	Heterogeneous across strata	Homogeneous across clusters

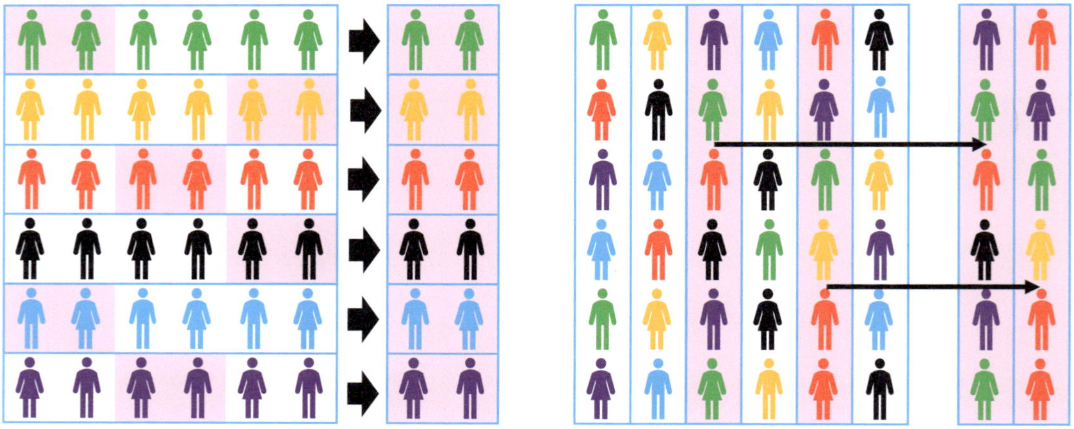

Fig. 5.11 Comparison of stratified random sampling and cluster random sampling processes

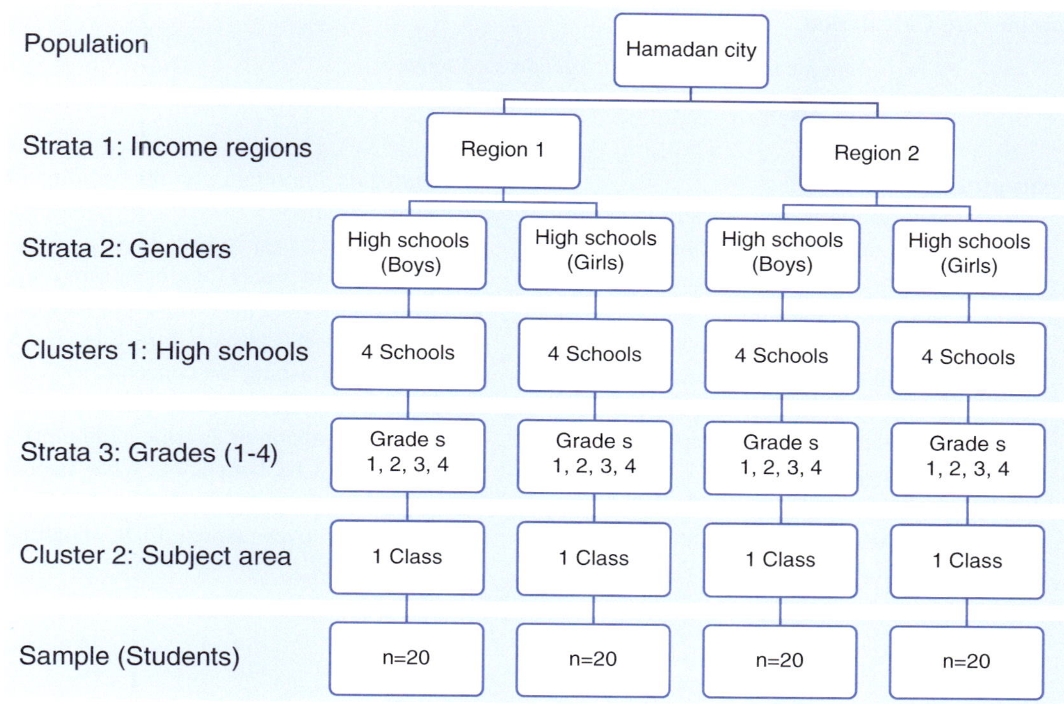

Fig. 5.12 Stratified cluster sampling design for smoking prevalence study

- Stratified sampling is like dividing a cake into layers (strata) and taking a slice from each layer.
- Cluster sampling is like dividing a cake into pieces (clusters) and selecting a few whole pieces.

5.10 Stratified Cluster Random Sampling

It is possible to combine stratified random sampling and cluster random sampling within a single study. For example, researchers investigating the prevalence of smoking among high school students in Hamadan City, Iran, employed a multistage sampling design, as illustrated in Fig. 5.12. The process included the following steps: [72]

1. Strata 1: The city was divided into high-income and low-income regions. Both regions (strata) were included in the sample.
2. Strata 2: Each region was further divided by gender, including both boys and girls. Both genders were included in the sample.
   - Cluster 1: From several boy and girl high schools, only four schools (clusters) were randomly selected from the available options.
3. Strata 3: Within each selected high school, students were stratified by educational grade (first to fourth grades), and all four grades (strata) were included in the sample.
   - Clusters 2: Within each grade, a single subject area (e.g., math) was randomly selected from the available subjects (clusters).
4. Finally, 20 students were randomly selected from each of these stratum-cluster categories.

Sample Size Calculation

$$\text{Sample size} = 2\,\text{regions} \times 2\,\text{genders} \times 4\,\text{schools} \times 4\,\text{grades} \times 1\,\text{class} \times 20\,\text{students} = 1280\,\text{students}$$

Conceptual Questions

1. What are the primary goals of stratified random sampling and cluster random sampling? How do these goals influence the choice of sampling method in research?
2. Describe how populations are divided in stratified random sampling versus cluster random sampling. What are the implications of these different approaches for the representativeness of the sample?
3. Explain the concepts of internal homogeneity and external heterogeneity in the context of stratified and cluster sampling. Why are these characteristics important for the validity of the research findings?
4. How does the cake analogy (layers for stratified sampling and pieces for cluster sampling) help in understanding the differences between these two methods? Discuss how this visualization aids in grasping the concepts.
5. Provide examples of research scenarios where a combined approach of stratified and cluster sampling would be beneficial. What factors would lead researchers to choose this integrated method over using either sampling technique alone?

Randomization Techniques in Clinical Trials

6

Contents

6.1 Random Allocation

Description
Random allocation, also known as *randomization*, is a technique used to assign individuals or items to groups in research studies. It ensures that each participant has an *equal* chance of being placed in any particular group. This is essential in research, especially in clinical trials, as it minimizes *bias* and helps obtain reliable results. Randomization also helps control for potential *confounding* factors that could influence the study's outcome. Figure 6.1 illustrates several methods for random allocation, each with its own advantages [2, 49].

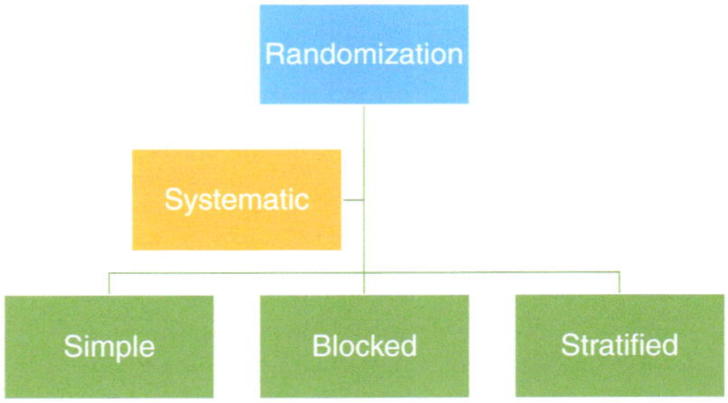

Fig. 6.1 Approaches to random allocation

J. Poorolajal, *Illustrated Epidemiology*, https://doi.org/10.1007/978-981-96-9566-9_6

Conceptual Questions

1. What is random allocation, and why is it a critical component of research design, particularly in clinical trials? Discuss how it contributes to the validity of study results.
2. Explain how random allocation assists in controlling for confounding factors. Why is it important to account for these factors in the analysis of study outcomes?
3. Discuss the significance of ensuring that each participant has an equal chance of being placed in any group. How does this principle enhance the reliability of the study findings?

6.2 Systematic Allocation

Description

Systematic allocation is a research method that assigns participants to groups using a predefined order. In this approach, participants are assigned based on a characteristic that follows a *predictable* sequence, such as:

- Date of admission
- Hospital or clinic record number
- Availability of the intervention
- Odd or even date of birth
- Patient's initials

While systematic allocation offers a way to distribute participants, it is *not* an acceptable randomization method [49]. This is because the assignment sequence can be easily predicted. Consequently, researchers or participants might be able to anticipate which treatment someone will receive, potentially introducing bias.

Advantages

1. Simplicity: Systematic randomization is straightforward to implement. Researchers can easily follow a defined procedure to select participants, making it user-friendly.
2. Time-efficient: This method can save time compared to simple random sampling, as it requires less effort in generating random numbers and can quickly produce a sample.
3. Even distribution: Systematic randomization can help ensure that the sample is evenly distributed across the population, reducing the risk of clustering that might occur in simple random sampling.

Disadvantages

1. Predictability: Systematic random allocation might allow for predictability if the allocation pattern (e.g., every fourth participant) is transparent. This could lead participants or investigators to manipulate the enrollment process to influence group assignments, potentially introducing selection bias.
2. Less true randomness: Systematic allocation is not fully random because once the starting point and interval are set, subsequent selections are determined. This reduced randomness can increase the risk of selection bias and affect the internal validity and statistical assumptions of the study.

Example

Imagine a hypothetical study investigating the effectiveness of a new pain medication compared to a standard pain medication. Researchers decide to use systematic allocation based on the date of admission, as illustrated in Fig. 6.2:

- Every patient admitted on an odd-numbered day (first, third, fifth, etc.) would be assigned to receive the new medication (drug A).
- Every patient admitted on an even-numbered day (second, fourth, sixth, etc.) would be assigned to receive the standard medication (drug B).

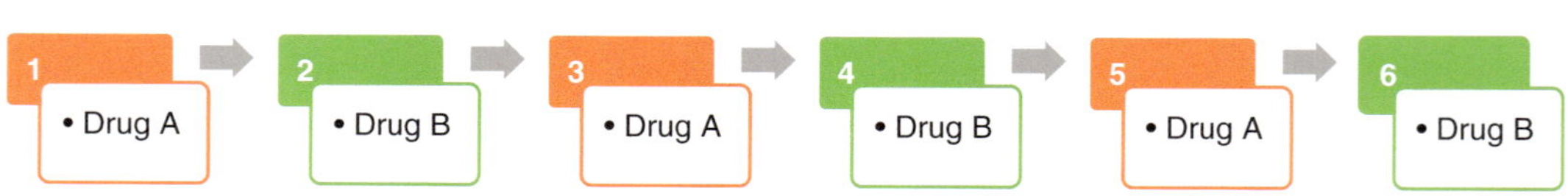

Fig. 6.2 Systematic allocation process

While this method may seem like a fair way to distribute participants, it has a significant flaw. Anyone involved in the study, including researchers and patients who know their admission date, could potentially guess which medication they will receive. This could introduce bias into the results.

Conceptual Questions

1. What is systematic allocation, and how does it differ from random allocation? Discuss the key characteristics that define systematic allocation as a method for assigning participants to groups.
2. Why is systematic allocation not considered an acceptable randomization method? Discuss how the predictability of the assignment sequence can introduce bias into the study results.
3. Provide examples of research scenarios where systematic allocation might be an appropriate choice despite its limitations. What factors would lead researchers to select this method?

6.3 Simple Random Allocation

Description

Simple random allocation is the most basic method for assigning participants to groups by chance. In this method, each participant has an *equal* probability of being assigned to any group, and this assignment is *independent* of any other factors, including the order in which participants are enrolled in the study [7, 49]. Figure 6.3 illustrates various methods of simple random allocation. This method works best with larger sample sizes, as smaller sample sizes increase the likelihood of group imbalance. For example, with a sample of 200 participants, the probability of imbalances in sampling fractions such as 55%|45%, 60%|40%, 65%|35%, and 70%|30% is relatively low (16%), very low (1%), negligible (0%), and nearly zero (0%), respectively [49].

Advantages

1. Equal probability: Every participant has an equal chance of being assigned to any group, minimizing selection bias and enhancing the comparability of the sample.

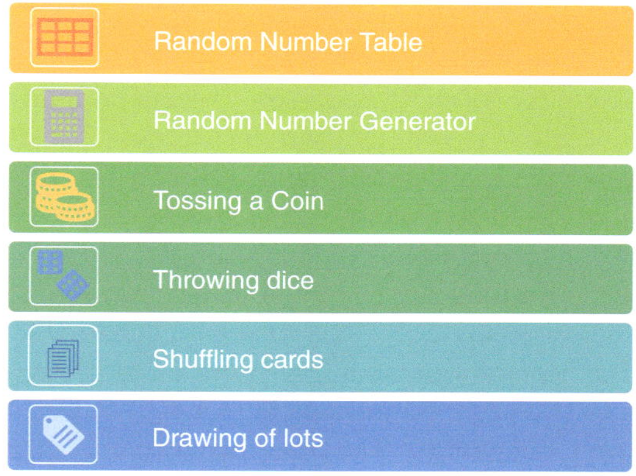
Random Number Table
Random Number Generator
Tossing a Coin
Throwing dice
Shuffling cards
Drawing of lots

Fig. 6.3 Simple random allocation methods

2. Simplicity: The method is straightforward to understand and implement, making it accessible for researchers and participants.
3. Statistical validity: Simple random allocation supports the validity of statistical analyses, as it ensures that groups are comparable at the outset of the study.
4. Flexibility: This method can be applied to various study designs and is suitable for different types of interventions and outcomes.

Disadvantages

1. Potential imbalance: Random allocation can lead to imbalances in group sizes or characteristics, especially in smaller samples, which may affect the statistical power.
2. Lack of control over group composition: Simple random allocation does not allow researchers to control for specific variables or characteristics, which may be important for certain studies.

Random Number Table

This method involves using a random number table, which can be found online or in statistics textbooks. A specific rule is established to interpret the numbers, such as even numbers indicating a new medication and odd numbers indicating standard treatment. Starting at a random point in the table, numbers are read sequentially, and each participant is assigned to a treatment group based on the predefined rule.

Example
A randomized controlled trial was conducted to assess the effect of educating mothers on injury prevention among children aged under 5 years using the health belief model (HBM). The randomization method involved selecting four local health centers from a total of 41, with two designated for the intervention group and two for the control group, utilizing a random number table. The centers were numbered from 01 to 41, and four two-digit numbers were randomly selected from this range. The first two centers were assigned to the intervention group, and the next two to the control group [73].

Random Number Generator
A computer program generates a random number for each participant, typically ranging from 1 to 2 for two groups, or from 1 to 3 for three groups, and so on. This number determines the treatment group assignment, with 1 representing the new medication, 2 representing the standard treatment, and so on.

Example
In the randomized double-blinded placebo-controlled pilot study assessing the effect of probiotics on nutritional absorption capacities in healthy children, a total of 40 pediatric patients aged 14 to 18 years were enrolled and randomly allocated into two groups: a treated group and a placebo group, with 20 participants in each. The randomization was conducted using a computerized random number generator, ensuring that all investigators remained blind to the treatment assignments [74].

Tossing a Coin
This method is useful for assigning participants to two groups. "Heads" corresponds to one treatment group (e.g., new treatment) and "tails" to the other (e.g., standard treatment). For each enrolled participant, flip a fair coin, and the outcome determines their treatment group.

Throwing Dice
This method can be adapted for more than two groups. Each possible outcome of the die roll is assigned to a specific treatment group (e.g., 1–3 = new medication, 4–6 = standard treatment). Roll the die for each enrolled participant, and the number rolled determines their treatment group.

Shuffling Cards
This method can be adapted for two or more groups. Half of the cards are marked for one treatment group (e.g., red for new treatment) and the other half for another group (e.g., black for standard treatment). Shuffle the deck thoroughly, and then draw a card from the top of the deck for each enrolled participant. The color of the cards determines their treatment group.

Drawing Lots
This method can be adapted for two or more groups. To prepare, create identical slips of paper, with half labeled for one treatment (e.g., new treatment) and the other half for the other (e.g., standard treatment). Fold the slips and place them in a container. Then, for each enrolled participant, draw a slip of paper, and the label will determine their treatment group.

Example
In the study examining the effects of kneeling posture on chest compression during cardiopulmonary resuscitation (CPR) in males, a self-controlled repeated-measures design was employed. Eighteen participants, all holding a qualified first-aid certificate, were recruited to perform CPR in three different kneeling postures: farthest, self-adjusted, and nearest. The order of the postures was randomized by drawing lots, ensuring that each participant experienced all three postures in a random sequence [75].

Conceptual Questions
1. What is simple random allocation, and how does it ensure that each participant has an equal probability of being assigned to any group? Discuss the independence of this method from other factors.
2. Why does simple random allocation work best with larger sample sizes? Discuss the implications of group imbalance in smaller

samples and how it can affect study outcomes.

3. Explain how a random number table can be used for simple random allocation. What steps must researchers follow to ensure proper assignment using this method?
4. How does a random number generator facilitate simple random allocation? What are the advantages of using technology in this process compared to traditional methods?
5. Discuss the use of a coin toss for assigning participants to two groups. What are the limitations of this method, especially in larger studies?
6. How can throwing dice or shuffling cards be adapted for studies with more than two groups? Provide examples of how these methods can be implemented in practice.
7. Describe the process of drawing lots for random allocation. What are the key considerations to ensure that this method is executed fairly and without bias?

6.4 Blocked Random Allocation

Description

Blocked randomization is a technique used in clinical trials to improve the balance of treatment groups, particularly in studies with smaller sample sizes. It achieves this by dividing the total number of participants into small blocks. Within each block, participants are randomly assigned to the various treatment arms. This method helps to minimize bias by ensuring that treatment groups have similar numbers of participants throughout the study, even if enrollment is staggered [49].

Table 6.1 illustrates a hypothetical randomized controlled trial involving 24 participants. Blocked randomization will divide them into six blocks of four participants each. Within each block, two participants will be randomly assigned to receive drug A, while the other two will receive drug B. The order of assignment for drugs A and B varies randomly within each block. For example, as shown in Table 6.1, the order in the first block might be B, A, A, and B, while in the second block, it could be A, B, B, A, and so on. This approach ensures that each treatment group has a similar number of participants, regardless of the order in which they are enrolled.

To implement this process, we will prepare four sheets of paper: two labeled with the name of the intervention and two labeled with the name of the control. These sheets will be pooled together and placed in a container. Participants will be assigned to either the intervention or control group by randomly drawing one paper sheet from the container at a time, without replacement, for each participant. Once all four sheets have been drawn, they will be returned to the container, and the drawing process will be repeated for each subsequent group of four participants until the desired sample size is reached.

Table 6.2 illustrates a hypothetical randomized controlled trial with a larger sample size. In this scenario, 56 eligible participants are divided into six blocks of nine participants each. This setup supports a three-arm study, where one-third of participants in each block are randomly assigned to receive drug A, drug B, or drug C.

To achieve this, we will prepare nine sheets of paper: three labeled "Intervention 1," three labeled "Intervention 2," and three labeled "Control." These sheets will be pooled together and placed in a container. Participants will be assigned to either the intervention groups or the control group by randomly drawing one paper

Table 6.1 Blocked randomization in a hypothetical two-arm trial (24 participants, six blocks of four)

Block 1		Block 2		Block 3		Block 4		Block 5		Block 6	
No.	Drug	No.	Drug	No.	Drug	No.	Drug	No.	Drug	No.	Drug
1	B	5	A	9	B	13	B	17	A	21	A
2	A	6	B	10	A	14	B	18	A	22	B
3	A	7	B	11	B	15	A	19	B	23	A
4	B	8	A	12	A	16	A	20	B	24	B

Table 6.2 Blocked randomization in a hypothetical three-arm trial (54 participants, six blocks of nine)

Block 1		Block 2		Block 3		Block 4		Block 5		Block 6	
No.	Drug	No.	Drug	No.	Drug	No.	Drug	No.	Drug	No.	Drug
1	B	10	A	19	C	28	B	37	A	46	C
2	A	11	B	20	A	29	A	38	C	47	A
3	C	12	C	21	B	30	C	39	B	48	B
4	C	13	B	22	A	31	C	40	B	49	B
5	B	14	A	23	C	32	A	41	C	50	C
6	A	15	C	24	B	33	B	42	A	51	A
7	C	16	C	25	C	34	B	43	C	52	C
8	B	17	A	26	A	35	C	44	B	53	B
9	A	18	B	27	B	36	A	45	A	54	A

sheet from the container at a time, without replacement, for each participant. Once all nine sheets have been drawn, they will be returned to the container, and the drawing process will be repeated for each subsequent group of nine participants until the desired sample size is achieved.

Advantages

1. Balance across groups: Blocked randomization ensures that each treatment group has a similar number of participants, thereby reducing the risk of group imbalances.
2. Improved statistical power: The increased balance in group sizes can enhance the statistical power of the study, making it easier to detect treatment effects.
3. Control for time-related biases: In studies with temporal recruitment, block randomization ensures that treatment groups are balanced across time, preventing bias from temporal trends.
4. Flexibility in block size: Researchers can adjust block sizes to match the study's sample size, providing greater control over group allocation.
5. Flexibility in design: Block randomization can be adapted for various trial designs and is particularly useful in studies with small sample sizes.

Disadvantages

1. Predictability: If the block size is known, it may lead to predictability in treatment assignment, potentially introducing bias if participants or researchers can anticipate the next allocation.
2. Potential for unequal group sizes: If the total sample size is not a multiple of the block size, it can result in unequal group sizes in the final sample, potentially affecting the analysis.

Example 1

Researchers aimed to investigate the effects of intravenous sodium valproate compared to dexamethasone on acute migraine headaches [76]. They randomly assigned 86 eligible patients to two groups using a blocked randomization method. To accomplish this, they prepared four slips of paper: two marked "V" for valproate and two marked "D" for dexamethasone. These slips were mixed, placed in a container, and drawn one at a time without replacement until all four slips were selected. This process was repeated until all 86 patients were enrolled, resulting in two groups of 43 patients each.

Example 2

In another study, researchers aimed to assess the effect of topical sucralfate and clindamycin compared to placebo on post-tonsillectomy pain in children [77]. They randomly assigned 110 eligible patients to three groups using a blocked randomization method. To do this, they prepared six slips of paper: two labeled "S" for sucralfate, two labeled "C" for clindamycin, and two labeled "P" for placebo. The slips were mixed, placed in a container, and drawn one at a time without replacement until all six slips were selected. This process was repeated until they reached the target sample size of 110 patients, resulting in three groups of 37, 36, and 37 patients, respectively.

Conceptual Questions

1. What is blocked randomization, and why is it used in clinical trials? Discuss how this method helps improve the balance of treatment groups, particularly in studies with smaller sample sizes.
2. Describe the process of blocked randomization. How are participants divided into blocks, and how are assignments made within each block?
3. What are the advantages of using blocked randomization compared to simple random allocation? How does it help minimize bias and ensure balanced treatment groups?
4. How does the overall sample size affect the size of each block and the number of treatment groups in a study? What implications does this have for researchers when planning their trials?
5. Provide examples of other research scenarios where blocked randomization would be an appropriate choice. What factors would lead researchers to select this method over other randomization techniques?

6.5 Stratified Random Allocation

Description

The stratified random allocation method is employed when known factors, such as age, gender, disease severity, medication use, and comorbidities, may influence outcomes, as depicted in Fig. 6.4. This figure shows a study with 140 participants divided into two gender strata: 80 males and 60 females. Each gender group is further stratified by age, with males categorized into 50 young and 30 old and females into 40 young and 20 old. Randomization is then applied within these strata to create a random sample. This method ensures that both gender and age are considered in the allocation process, promoting balanced representation in the treatment groups [2, 49].

Stratification aims to minimize variability among participants within each subgroup (within-strata) while maximizing variability between different subgroups (between-strata). This targeted method helps prevent imbalances in the distribution of important factors (covariates) that could affect the study's results.

Advantages

1. Enhanced representativeness: By ensuring that key subgroups (e.g., gender, age) are adequately represented, stratified randomization improves the generalizability of study results.
2. Reduced variability: This method helps control for confounding variables, leading to more precise estimates of treatment effects by minimizing variability within treatment groups.
3. Increased statistical power: With balanced representation across strata, the study may have greater statistical power to detect differences between treatment groups.

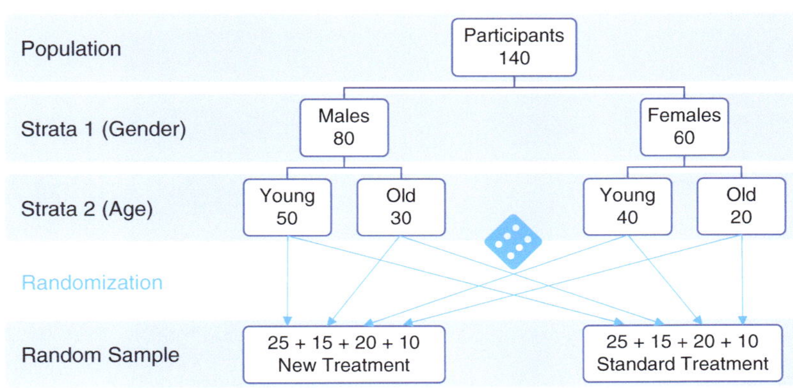

Fig. 6.4 Stratified random allocation by gender and age

4. Tailored analysis: Researchers can analyze outcomes within specific strata, allowing for more detailed insights into how different subgroups respond to treatments.

Disadvantages

1. Complexity in design: Stratified randomization can complicate the study design and implementation, requiring careful planning to define strata and manage randomization.
2. Risk of overstratification: Too many strata can lead to difficulties in randomization and analysis, especially if some strata have very few participants, potentially complicating the interpretation of results.

Example

As illustrated in Fig. 6.5, the clinical trial comparing the effects of heparin, reteplase, and taurolock in preventing thrombosis in hemodialysis catheters employed a stratified random allocation method to assign patients to five groups: control, heparin 50, heparin 1000, reteplase, and taurolock. Patients were stratified based on characteristics such as age, gender, and duration of dialysis, resulting in eight strata. Within each stratum, patients were randomly assigned to one of the five treatment groups using a randomized block permutation method to ensure balanced distribution. To enhance the study's rigor, a triple-blind design was implemented, keeping patients, thrombosis assessors, and statistical analysts unaware of the assigned interventions. This comprehensive randomization approach aimed to minimize bias and validate the findings regarding thrombosis incidence across the different treatment groups [78].

Conceptual Questions

1. What is stratified random allocation, and why is it used in research studies? Discuss how this method addresses known factors that might influence study outcomes.
2. Describe how participants are divided into strata in stratified random allocation. What factors (e.g., age, gender) are typically considered, and why are they important for the study design?
3. Discuss how stratification aims to minimize variability within subgroups while maximizing variability between different subgroups. Why is this balance important for the validity of the study findings?
4. What are the advantages of using stratified random allocation compared to simple random allocation? How does it enhance the representativeness of the sample?

6.6 Cluster Random Allocation

Description

A cluster refers to a group or collection of individuals or units that share certain characteristics, such as geographical location, institutions (like schools, hospitals, clinics, health centers, or workplaces), or other natural groupings. Cluster random allocation is a method used in randomized controlled trials (RCTs) where groups or clusters of participants, rather than individual

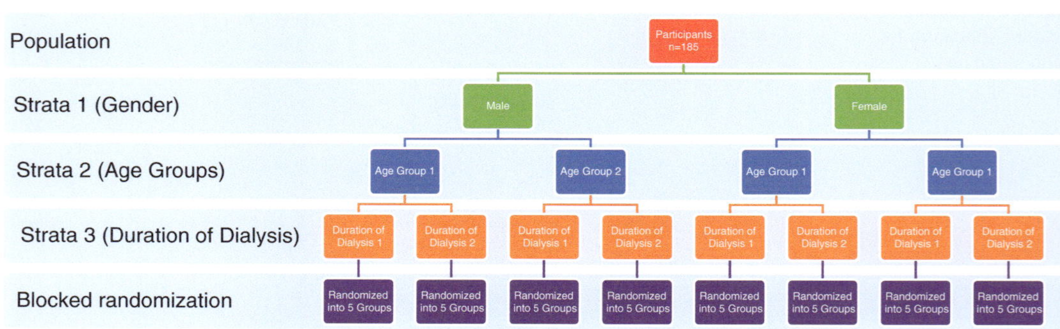

Fig. 6.5 Stratified random allocation by gender, age, and duration of dialysis

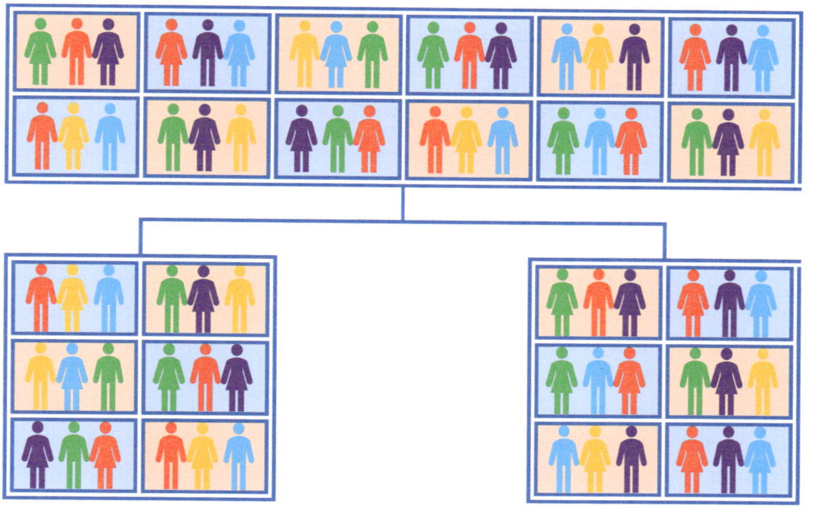

Fig. 6.6 Cluster random allocation

participants, are randomly assigned to different treatment or intervention groups, as shown in Fig. 6.6. This approach is particularly useful in situations where individual randomization is impractical or could lead to contamination between groups. In cluster random allocation, entire groups (or clusters) of participants are assigned to receive either the intervention or the control treatment.

Advantages

1. Reduced contamination: By randomizing clusters, the risk of contamination is minimized, particularly in educational interventions. This approach helps prevent participants in the control group from inadvertently becoming aware of the educational context through interactions with the intervention group.
2. Practicality: Cluster randomization is often more feasible for community-based interventions or public health studies, where it may be logistically simpler to implement an intervention at the group level.

Disadvantages

1. Statistical complexity: Analyzing data from cluster-randomized trials can be more complex than from individually randomized trials, as outcomes from participants within the same cluster may be correlated.
2. Increased sample size requirements: Cluster randomization often requires a larger sample size to achieve adequate statistical power, as the variability within clusters can reduce the effective sample size.

Example 1

As illustrated in Fig. 6.7, in a hypothetical public health study aimed at reducing childhood obesity, researchers utilized cluster random allocation by selecting ten elementary schools as clusters within a district. These schools were randomly assigned to either an intervention group, which implemented a new nutrition and physical activity program, or a control group that continued with their standard curriculum. The intervention included workshops for parents, modifications to the school lunch menu, and increased physical activity opportunities for students. At the end of the school year, data on outcomes such as changes in body mass index (BMI), dietary habits, and physical activity levels were collected and analyzed to compare the effectiveness of the program between the intervention and control schools, accounting for the clustering effect.

Example 2

A cluster randomized controlled trial was conducted to assess the effectiveness of an organ donation intervention in increasing the number of signed donor cards among employees. A total of

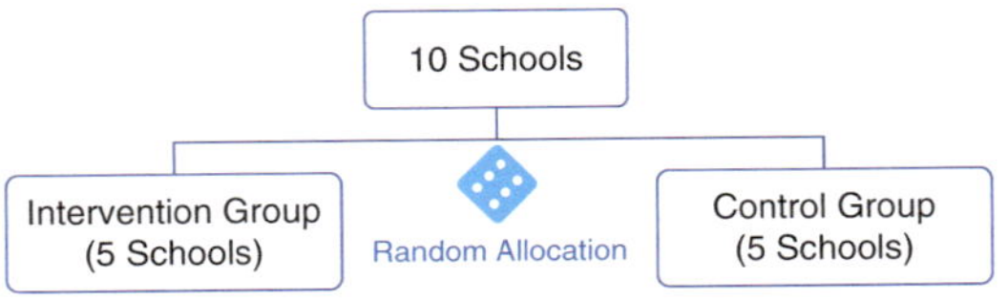

Fig. 6.7 Randomized cluster design: allocation of ten schools to intervention (five schools) and control (five schools) groups

28 offices were selected as clusters, with every two offices matched based on their occupational type and profession. From each matched pair, one office was randomly assigned to the intervention group, which received a multicomponent program involving training and family engagement, while the other office served as the control group. The study aimed for a sample size of 324 participants (162 in each group). Data were collected using a self-administered questionnaire at multiple time points, revealing a significantly higher proportion of participants in the intervention group who signed donor cards compared to the control group (73.2% vs. 17.9%), along with notable improvements in various psychosocial constructs related to organ donation [79].

Conceptual Questions

1. What is cluster random allocation, and in what scenarios is it particularly advantageous compared to individual randomization?
2. Explain how cluster random allocation reduces the risk of contamination between intervention and control groups. Additionally, can you provide an example of a situation where contamination might occur in an individually randomized trial?
3. Why do cluster randomized trials often require a larger sample size than individually randomized trials?

Matching Methods in Epidemiological Studies

7

Contents

7.1 Matching

Description
Matching is the process of selecting controls that are similar to the cases in certain characteristics believed to influence the outcome of interest, such as age, sex, socioeconomic status, or other confounding variables. The goal of matching is to ensure that the control group is *comparable* to the case group, which helps to minimize the impact of confounding factors and improve the validity of the study's findings. Matching is done particularly in case-control studies but can also be used in cohort studies and clinical trials [7, 8, 80].

As illustrated in Fig. 7.1, there are two main approaches to matching in epidemiological studies: frequency matching and individual matching. We will discuss the types of matching later in this chapter.

Advantages
1. Control of confounding variables: Matching helps to eliminate or reduce the influence of confounding variables, making it easier to identify the true effect of the exposure on the outcome.
2. Improved comparability: By matching participants on key characteristics (e.g., age, sex, socioeconomic status), researchers create more comparable groups, enhancing the validity of the study findings.
3. Increased statistical power: With reduced variability within matched groups, the statistical power of the study can increase, allowing for more precise estimates of the effect.

Disadvantages
1. Complexity in design: Designing a matched study can be complex and time-consuming, requiring careful selection of matching criteria and participants.
2. Loss of generalizability: The results may not be generalizable to the broader population if the matched characteristics are too restrictive or specific.
3. Difficulty in analysis: Analyzing matched data can be more complicated than unmatched data, often requiring specialized statistical techniques.

J. Poorolajal, *Illustrated Epidemiology*, https://doi.org/10.1007/978-981-96-9566-9_7

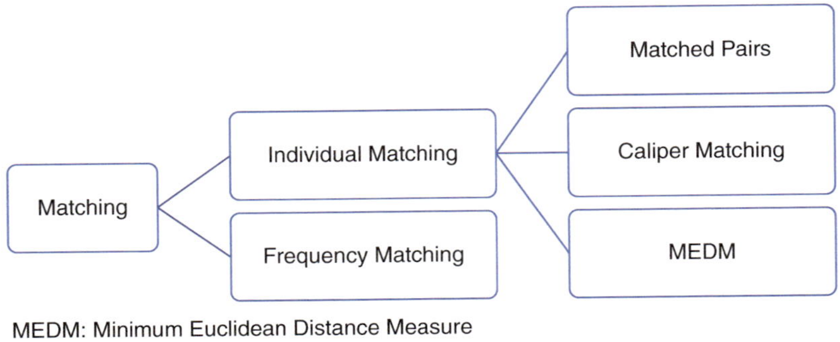

Fig. 7.1 Classification of different matching techniques

4. Limited to known confounders: Matching only accounts for confounders that are known and measured; unmeasured confounders can still bias results.

Conceptual Questions

1. What is matching in the context of epidemiological studies, and why is it important? Discuss how matching helps to control for confounding variables and improve the validity of study findings.
2. What are confounding factors, and how does matching help to mitigate their impact on study outcomes? Discuss the importance of identifying relevant confounders before matching.
3. What are some potential limitations or challenges associated with matching in research studies?
4. Provide examples of research scenarios where matching would be particularly beneficial. What factors would lead researchers to choose matching as a technique over other methods of controlling for confounding variables?

7.2 Frequency Matching

Description

In frequency matching, the overall frequency distribution of the matching variables is equalized between the case and control groups, without necessarily matching individual subjects one-to-one. The goal is to *balance* the *distribution* of the matching variables between the two groups, rather than creating matched pairs.

By matching on key characteristics, frequency matching helps control for potential confounders, allowing for a clearer assessment of the relationship between exposure and outcome. However, unlike one-to-one matching, frequency matching does not ensure that specific individuals in the case and control groups are directly comparable, which may obscure individual-level differences.

Frequency matching data does *not* require specific statistical tests tailored exclusively for matched designs, such as those used in one-to-one matching. Instead, researchers can analyze frequency-matched data using standard statistical techniques applicable to independent samples, as the focus is on the overall distribution of matched characteristics rather than individual pairings. This flexibility allows for the use of *common* statistical methods, such as independent t-test, logistic regression, or chi-square test, to assess associations between exposure and outcome while controlling for the matched characteristics. Consequently, frequency matching simplifies the analytical process, making it more accessible for researchers and facilitating the interpretation of results without the complexities associated with specialized matching analyses.

Example 1

Figure 7.2 illustrates a hypothetical frequency-matched case-control study in which cases and controls are matched on sex, age, smoking status, and color, which serves as a proxy for other confounding variables such as socioeconomic status or income levels. Importantly, individual subjects in the case and control groups are not matched one-to-one; rather, the overall distribution of these factors is balanced between the two groups.

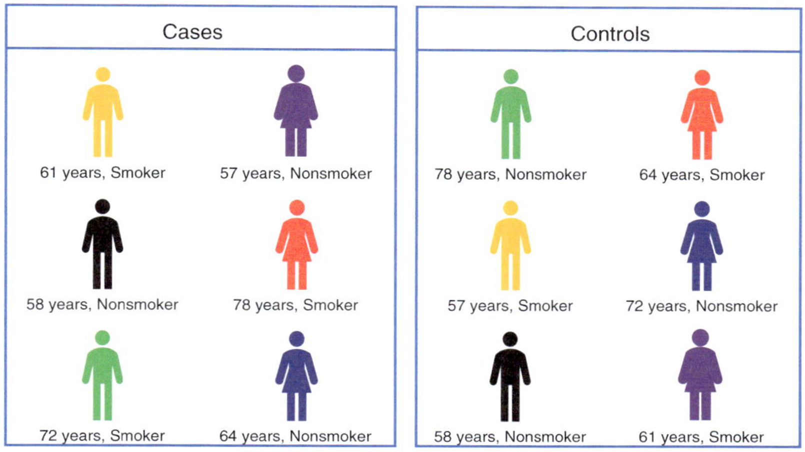

Fig. 7.2 Frequency-matched case-control study design

Example 2
A matched case-control study investigated the impact of maternal COVID-19 exposure on placental characteristics, involving 15 COVID-19 positive mothers and 36 negative mothers. The cases and controls were frequency matched by gestational age, race, maternal comorbidities, and delivery type to ensure comparability, resulting in no significant differences between the groups regarding demographic or clinical characteristics [81].

Synonyms
Frequency matching; Group matching

Conceptual Questions
1. Describe the process of frequency matching. How does this method ensure that the distribution of certain characteristics (e.g., age, sex) in the control group reflects that of the case group? Provide an example to illustrate this approach.
2. What statistical tests are commonly used to analyze frequency-matched data in case-control studies, and how do these differ from the tests used for analyzing data from individually matched studies?
3. What are the advantages of using frequency matching in epidemiological studies? How does it help to control for confounding variables while maintaining a larger pool of subjects?

7.3 Individual Matching

Description
In individual matching, each subject in the case group is matched one-to-one or one-to-many with subjects in the control group based on specific characteristics. This ensures that the case and control groups are well balanced on the matching variables.

Individual matching can be adapted for continuous variables. Finding exact matches on continuous variables like age can be challenging. *Caliper matching* addresses this by allowing a predefined range around the case's value. For example, if a case is 45 years old, controls within 3 years (42–48 years) might be considered acceptable matches.

Analyzing individual-matched data typically requires the use of specific statistical tests that account for the paired nature of the data. In an individual-matched case-control study, each case is paired with a control based on certain characteristics, which means that the observations are not independent. To properly analyze this type of data, researchers often employ statistical methods such as paired t-test, conditional logistic regression, or McNemar's test, which are designed to handle the dependencies created by the matching process. These methods allow for a more accurate assessment of the relationship between exposure and outcome by controlling for the matched characteristics at the individual level. While this approach provides robust insights into the associations being studied, it also necessitates a more complex analytical framework compared to frequency-matched designs, emphasizing the importance of using appropriate statistical techniques to account for the matched pairs.

Example 1

Figure 7.3 depicts a hypothetical matched case-control study where cases and controls are individually matched one-to-one on sex, age, smoking status, and color (used as a proxy to represent different socioeconomic groups or income levels). In this approach, for every individual with a particular sex, age, smoking status, and color in the case group, there is a corresponding subject with the same characteristics in the control group.

Example 2

A matched case-control study investigated the association between autism spectrum disorder (ASD) and maternal and perinatal risk factors in Hamadan, Iran, from November 2015 to May 2016. The study enrolled 41 children with ASD, for whom four controls were selected from the same hospital for each case, ensuring that controls were matched for sex, age, and birth year. In total, 41 ASD cases were compared with 164 matched controls. The analysis revealed significant associations between ASD and various maternal and perinatal risk factors, highlighting the need for further research through large prospective multicenter cohort studies to better understand these associations [82].

Synonyms

Individual-matched; Matched pairs; Exact matching

Conceptual Questions

1. Discuss the concept of individual matching. How does this method work, and what are the advantages and disadvantages compared to frequency matching? Provide an example of when individual matching might be preferred.
2. What are some potential limitations or challenges associated with individual matching? How might these limitations affect the validity of the study's findings?
3. Explain the concept of caliper matching as it applies to continuous variables. How does this method help researchers find acceptable matches when exact matches are difficult to obtain?
4. How does individual matching influence the statistical analysis of data in case-control studies? What statistical methods are typically used to account for the matched design?

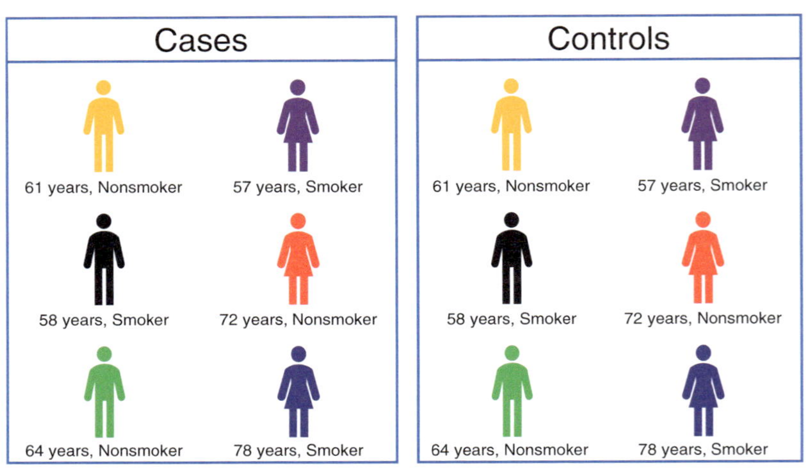

Fig. 7.3 Individual-matched case-control study design

7.4 Minimum Euclidean Distance Measure (MEDM)

Description

Matching on *multiple continuous* variables can be increasingly challenging with exact matching techniques. A solution to this problem is the minimum Euclidean distance measure (MEDM), which represents a specialized form of *individual* matching. MEDM identifies the control subject in a multidimensional space whose combined values across all matching variables are closest to those of the case, as determined by the shortest Euclidean distance. This approach allows for a more flexible and efficient matching process, enabling researchers to effectively pair cases with controls based on multiple continuous variables while maintaining the integrity of individual-level comparisons.

Example 1

Figure 7.4 illustrates a hypothetical matched case-control study where cases and controls are individually matched one-to-one on age and body mass index (BMI). However, finding control subjects with an exact match to corresponding cases in both age and BMI is nearly impossible. Based on the MEDM, every control subject in the two-dimensional space whose combined values on age and BMI are closest to a case will be considered its control.

Example 2

A matched case-control study utilized the MEDM for matching cases and controls based on several continuous variables. In this approach, each case was paired with two controls according to specific variables to minimize bias due to confounding. Matching was performed on categorical variables, such as sex and race, which required exact matches, as well as on continuous variables, such as age and systolic blood pressure, which were matched using the minimum Euclidean distance calculated from z-scores. In this study, which involved 91 cases and 182 controls, the researchers ensured that the age difference between cases and controls was minimal, with a maximum difference of 3 years for initial matches and 5 years for subsequent matches. This method allowed for close matching on multiple variables, enhancing the study's ability to control for confounding factors and providing clearer results [83].

Conceptual Questions

1. What is the minimum Euclidean distance measure (MEDM), and why is it used in matching cases and controls? Discuss how it addresses the challenges of matching on multiple continuous variables.
2. Describe the process of matching cases and controls using MEDM. How does the MEDM approach differ from traditional exact matching methods?
3. What are the advantages of using MEDM for matching in epidemiological studies? How does it enhance the feasibility and effectiveness of matching when dealing with multiple continuous variables?
4. Provide examples of research scenarios where MEDM would be particularly useful. What factors would lead researchers to choose this method over other matching techniques?

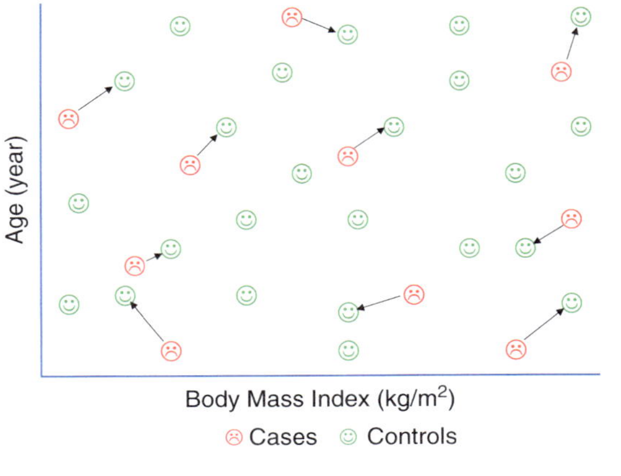

Fig. 7.4 Matching cases and controls using minimum Euclidean distance measure (MEDM)

8 Measures of Association in Epidemiology

Contents

8.1 Risk Ratio, Rate Ratio, Odds Ratio, and Risk Difference

These terms help quantify the relationship between an intervention (such as a drug) or exposure (such as a risk factor) and an outcome (such as a disease). They offer different perspectives, and the best choice depends on the study design and the type of outcome.

Consider a hypothetical prospective cohort study with 100 smokers and 100 nonsmokers. They are followed for 5 years to evaluate the impact of smoking on bronchitis. The results of this study are outlined in Table 8.1. Person-years represent the total follow-up time for all participants.

Risk Ratio

A risk ratio (RR) compares the probability of an outcome (e.g., bronchitis) occurring in the exposed group (e.g., smokers) to that in the unexposed group (e.g., nonsmokers). It is commonly used in cohort studies and randomized controlled trials, where participants are followed over time and categorized based on their exposure or intervention status. Since the risk ratio is obtained by dividing two probabilities (the probability of disease in the exposed group by the probability of disease in the unexposed group), it ranges from zero to positive infinity (0 to ∞).

- A risk ratio greater than 1 indicates that the exposed group has a higher risk of the outcome compared to the unexposed group.
- A risk ratio less than 1 suggests that the exposed group has a lower risk.
- A risk ratio of 1 signifies that the risk is equal for both groups.

$$\text{Risk ratio} = \frac{a / n_1}{c / n_2} = \frac{80 / 100}{40 / 100} = 2.0$$

A risk ratio of 2.0 indicates that smokers are twice as likely to experience bronchitis compared to nonsmokers.

Rate Ratio

The rate ratio is similar to the risk ratio, but instead of comparing simple risks, it compares the rates (events per unit of time) of the outcome between exposed and unexposed groups. Rate ratios are commonly used in follow-up studies such as cohort studies and randomized controlled trials. The interpretation of a rate ratio is similar

J. Poorolajal, *Illustrated Epidemiology*, https://doi.org/10.1007/978-981-96-9566-9_8

Table 8.1 Results of a hypothetical prospective cohort study

Groups	Bronchitis	No bronchitis	Total	Person-year
Smokers	80 a	20 b	100 n_1	425 py_1
Nonsmokers	40 c	60 d	100 n_2	472 py_2

to that of a risk ratio. Since the rate ratio is calculated by dividing two rates (the rate of disease in the exposed group by the rate of disease in the unexposed group), it ranges from zero to positive infinity (0 to ∞).

- A rate ratio greater than 1 indicates that the exposed group has a higher rate of the outcome compared to the unexposed group.
- A rate ratio less than 1 suggests that the exposed group has a lower rate.
- A rate ratio of 1 signifies that the rate is equal for both groups.

$$\text{Rate ratio} = \frac{a / \text{py}_1}{c / \text{py}_2} = \frac{80 / 425}{40 / 472} = 2.2$$

A rate ratio of 2.2 suggests that the rate of developing bronchitis in smokers is 2.2 times higher than in nonsmokers.

Odds Ratio

The odds ratio compares the odds (chance) of experiencing an outcome in the exposed group (e.g., smokers) to that in the unexposed group (e.g., nonsmokers). It is commonly used in case-control and cross-sectional studies but can also be applied in cohort studies and randomized controlled trials. Since the odds ratio is calculated by dividing the odds of disease in the exposed group by the odds of disease in the unexposed group, it ranges from zero to positive infinity (0 to ∞).

- An odds ratio greater than 1 indicates that the exposed group has higher odds of experiencing the outcome compared to the unexposed group.
- An odds ratio less than 1 suggests that the exposed group has lower odds of experiencing the outcome.
- An odds ratio of 1 indicates that the exposure has no effect on the odds of developing the outcome.

$$\text{Odds ratio} = \frac{a / b}{c / d} = \frac{ad}{bc} = \frac{80 \times 60}{20 \times 40} = 6.0$$

A result of 6.0 indicates that the chance of having bronchitis is six times greater in smokers compared to nonsmokers.

Risk Difference

The risk difference is the absolute difference in the risk (probability) of an outcome between the exposed and unexposed groups. It can be utilized in both cohort studies and randomized controlled trials. Since the risk difference is calculated by subtracting the risk of disease in the unexposed group from the risk of disease in the exposed group, it can range from negative one (−1) to positive one (+1).

- A positive risk difference indicates a higher risk in the exposed group.
- A negative risk difference suggests a lower risk in the exposed group.
- A risk difference of zero means the risk is the same for both groups.

$$\text{Risk difference} = (a / n_1) - (c / n_2) = 0.8 - 0.4 = 0.4 = 40\%$$

A result of 0.4 (or 40%) indicates that the risk of bronchitis in smokers is 40% higher than in nonsmokers.

Synonyms

Risk ratio; Relative risk

Rate ratio; Relative rate

Odds ratio; Relative odds

Risk difference; Attributable risk; Excess risk

Conceptual Questions

1. Define risk ratio, rate ratio, odds ratio, and risk difference. In what contexts are each of these measures most appropriately used? Discuss how the choice of measure can depend on the study design and type of outcome.
2. Interpret the risk ratio of 2.0 in the context of the study. What does this indicate about the likelihood of developing bronchitis among smokers compared to nonsmokers?
3. Explain the significance of the rate ratio of 2.2. How does this measure differ from the risk ratio, and why might researchers choose to use the rate ratio instead?
4. Describe how the odds ratio is calculated using the provided data. What does an odds ratio of 6.0 indicate about the odds of developing bronchitis for smokers compared to nonsmokers?
5. What does a risk difference of 0.4 (or 40%) signify in this study? How can this measure be useful in public health decision-making?

8.2 Probability Versus Odds

Probability

Probability is a measure of the likelihood of an event occurring. It is expressed as a number between 0 and 1, where 0 means the event is impossible and 1 means the event is certain.

Example: As shown in Fig. 8.1, the probability of developing the disease of interest is 10/30 or 33%.

$$\text{Probability} = \frac{\text{Disease}}{\text{Total sample}} = \frac{10}{30} = 0.33$$

Odds

Odds represent the ratio of the number of events to the number of nonevents. Unlike probability, odds can range from 0 to infinity, with 0 denoting impossibility and infinity representing certainty.

Example: As shown in Fig. 8.1, the odds of developing the disease of interest are 10/20 or 50%.

$$\text{Odds} = \frac{\text{Disease}}{\text{Non}-\text{disease}} = \frac{10}{20} = 0.50$$

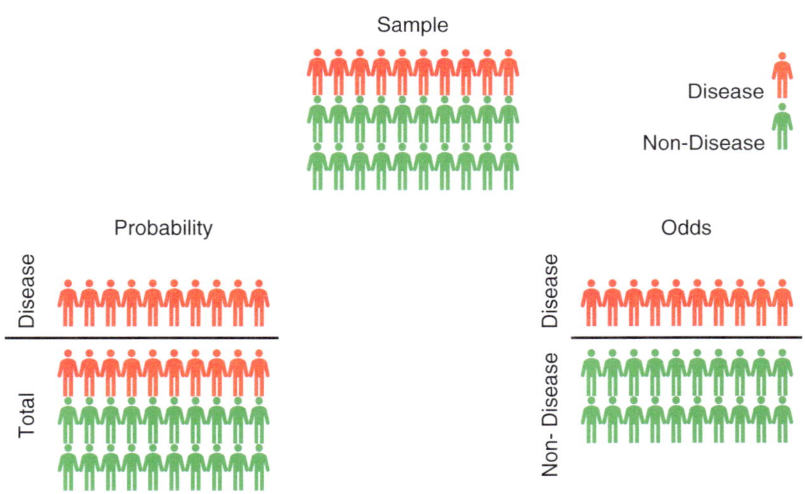

Fig. 8.1 Comparison of probability and odds

Converting Probability to Odds

To convert probability (P) to odds (O), use the following formula:

$$O = \frac{P}{1-P}$$

Example: If the probability of an event is $P = 0.33$:

$$\mathrm{O} = \frac{P}{1-P} = \frac{0.33}{1-0.33} = \frac{0.33}{0.67} = 0.50$$

Converting Odds to Probability

To convert odds (O) back to probability (P), use the following formula:

$$P = \frac{O}{1+O}$$

Example: If the odds of an event are $O = 0.50$:

$$P = \frac{0.50}{1+0.50} = \frac{0.50}{1.50} = 0.33$$

Conceptual Questions

1. Define probability and odds. How do they differ in terms of their mathematical representation and interpretation? Provide examples to illustrate these differences.
2. Using the example provided, explain how to calculate the probability of developing the disease. What does a probability of 0.33 (or 33%) indicate about the likelihood of the event occurring?
3. Explain how to calculate the odds of developing the disease using the example provided. What does an odds of 0.50 (or 50%) signify in this context?
4. Discuss the mathematical relationship between probability and odds. How can one be converted into the other? Provide the formulas for converting probability to odds and vice versa.

Errors, Biases, Confounding, and Interaction in Epidemiological Research

9

Contents

9.1 Errors in Epidemiological Studies

Description

Errors in epidemiological studies can have a significant impact on the validity and reliability of research findings. As illustrated in Fig. 9.1, these errors can be categorized into three main categories [7, 8].

Random Errors

Random error refers to unpredictable variations in measurements that occur due to inherent fluctuations in the measurement process, leading to results that scatter around the true value without a consistent pattern. It affects the *precision* of study results and can be minimized by using larger sample sizes.

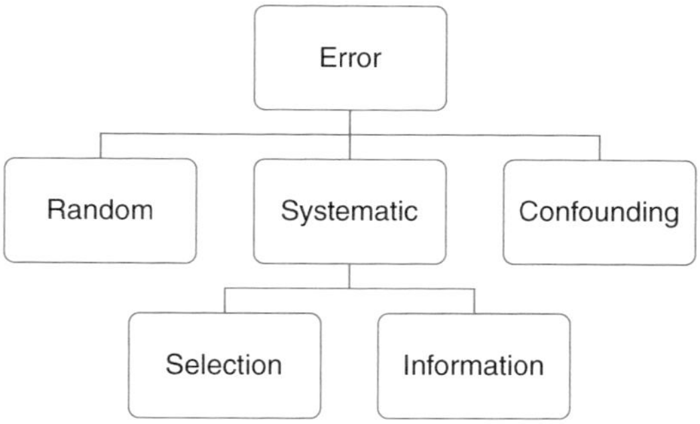

Fig. 9.1 Errors in epidemiological studies

Systematic Errors

Systematic error, or *bias*, is a consistent deviation from the true value that impacts the *accuracy* of results. It often arises from flaws in data collection, analysis, or interpretation, such as issues

J. Poorolajal. *Illustrated Epidemiology*, https://doi.org/10.1007/978-981-96-9566-9_9

with study design or measurement tools, which can lead to incorrect conclusions that *cannot* be corrected by increasing sample size. Systematic error is typically divided into two subcategories:

- *Selection bias*, arising from biases in participant selection that can lead to unrepresentative samples
- *Information bias*, resulting from inaccuracies in data collection that can distort findings

Confounding
Confounding error occurs when an external variable influences both the independent and dependent variables, distorting the observed relationship between them, making it appear stronger, weaker, or even in the opposite direction than it truly is.

Conceptual Questions
1. What are the main types of errors that can occur in epidemiological studies? Discuss how these errors can impact the validity and reliability of research findings.
2. What measures can researchers take to minimize errors in epidemiological studies? Discuss best practices for study design, data collection, and analysis to enhance the validity of findings.
3. How can understanding these categories of errors improve the design and execution of future epidemiological studies?
4. Why is it important to distinguish between different types of errors when evaluating the validity of epidemiological studies?

9.2 Random Error Versus Systematic Error

Random Error
Random error occurs due to chance variations in measurements. Even when performed carefully, repeated measurements of the same item will yield slightly different results. This type of error affects the *precision* of measurements. As illustrated in Fig. 9.2, random error tends to decrease as the sample size increases [7, 84].

Example 1: Random Error
In a study examining blood pressure in a population, random error can occur due to chance variations in the individuals selected for the sample and the measurement process itself. For example, a small sample might overrepresent individuals with naturally higher or lower blood pressure compared to the true population average. Additionally, factors like variations in time of day, recent physical activity, caffeine intake, or even slight

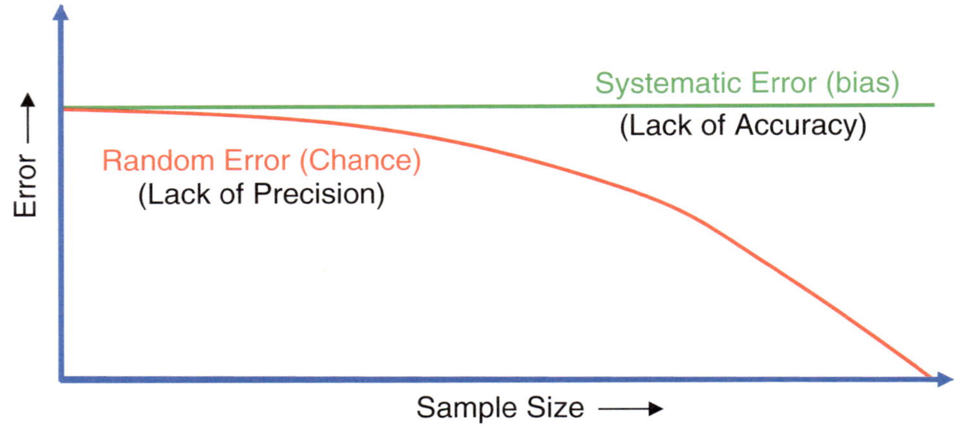

Fig. 9.2 Impact of an increase in sample size on random error and systematic error

inconsistencies in the blood pressure cuff placement can introduce random fluctuations in the measured blood pressure values. However, as the sample size increases, the impact of these random variations tends to diminish. A larger sample is more likely to include a representative range of individuals and minimize the influence of these chance occurrences, leading to a more accurate and precise estimate of the true population mean blood pressure.

Example 2: Random Error
When estimating the prevalence of diabetes in a population, the sample size plays a crucial role in determining the precision of the estimate due to random error. For instance, in a small sample of 50 individuals, random fluctuations can lead to significant variability in prevalence estimates. If 20 out of 50 are found to have diabetes, the estimated prevalence would be 40%, whereas a different sample might yield only five out of 50, resulting in a prevalence of 10%. As the sample size increases, the impact of these random fluctuations diminishes. A larger sample is more likely to be representative of the true population, meaning it will include a wider range of individuals with varying diabetes status. This leads to a more stable and accurate estimate of the true prevalence. In essence, with larger samples, the estimates tend to cluster more closely around the true population prevalence, reducing the influence of random chance and providing more reliable results.

Systematic Error
Systematic error (or bias) consistently shifts measurements in one direction, either overestimating or underestimating the true value. This type of error impacts the *accuracy* of results. As illustrated in Fig. 9.2, unlike random error, systematic error is not reduced by increasing sample size [7, 84].

Example 3: Systematic Error
In a study examining BMI in a population, systematic error can occur if the scale used to measure weight consistently provides inaccurate readings. For example, if the scale consistently adds 2 kilograms to the true weight of each participant, it will lead to a systematic overestimation of weight across the entire sample. This, in turn, will systematically overestimate BMI (since BMI is calculated as weight divided by height squared). Increasing the sample size in this scenario will not correct the error; the BMI calculations will still be systematically biased due to the consistent error in weight measurement. This highlights how systematic errors, unlike random errors, can persist even with large sample sizes and can significantly impact the accuracy of study findings.

Example 4: Systematic Error
If a study estimating socioeconomic status (SES) relies solely on an online survey, it may introduce selection bias. Individuals with higher socioeconomic status are more likely to have regular Internet access, own computers, and possess the digital literacy skills necessary to complete online surveys. Conversely, individuals with lower socioeconomic status may have limited or no Internet access, lack access to computers, or face language or literacy barriers that prevent them from participating in online surveys. This results in an overrepresentation of individuals with higher SES and an underrepresentation of those with lower SES in the study sample, leading to a biased and inaccurate estimation of the true distribution of SES in the population, regardless of the sample size.

The key differences between random error and systematic error are illustrated in Table 9.1.

Conceptual Questions
1. Define random error and systematic error. What are the key characteristics that

Table 9.1 Key differences between random error and systematic error

Feature	Random error	Systematic error
Consistency	Inconsistent with no specific direction	Consistent with one direction
Impact	Primarily reduces precision	Primarily reduces accuracy
Sample size	Decreases with larger sample size	Does not change with sample size

distinguish these two types of errors from one another?
2. Explain how sample size influences random error and systematic error. Why does increasing the sample size help reduce random error but not systematic error?
3. Provide examples of situations where random error might occur in epidemiological studies. How can researchers identify and account for random error in their analyses?
4. What are the statistical implications of random error and systematic error in data analysis? How might each type of error affect the results of hypothesis testing and confidence intervals?

9.3 Random Error

Description

Random error refers to unpredictable fluctuations in measurements caused by chance, affecting the *precision* of results [84]. It can occur in any study and is typically reflected in the standard error (SE). A wider normal curve, as shown in Fig. 9.3, indicates a higher SE and thus more random error.

A higher SE suggests more variability or uncertainty in estimating a population parameter (e.g., the mean), implying greater random error in the sample estimate. Conversely, a lower SE indicates more precision in the sample mean and less random error.

It is important to note that standard error not only reflects *random error* but also the inherent *variability* in the data. SE depends on both the *variance* of the data and the *sample size*—larger samples typically lead to smaller SE, reducing the impact of random error.

Example

In a study estimating the prevalence of alcohol consumption, random error can occur due to variability in the selection of individuals. With a small sample size, there is a higher likelihood of disproportionate representation—for example, the sample might include more abstainers due to religious or health reasons, leading to an underestimation, or it might overrepresent frequent drinkers from social environments where alcohol is common, leading to an overestimation. However, as the sample size increases, the probability of such disproportionate representation decreases. Larger samples are more likely to include a balanced and representative mix of individuals with varying drinking habits, such as abstainers, moderate drinkers, and heavy drinkers. This improved representation reduces the influence of random fluctuations and results in a more reliable estimate of the true prevalence of alcohol consumption within the population.

Conceptual Questions

1. Explain how sample size influences random error. Why does increasing the sample size help reduce random error?
2. Provide examples of situations where random error might occur in epidemiological studies. How can researchers identify and account for random error in their analyses?

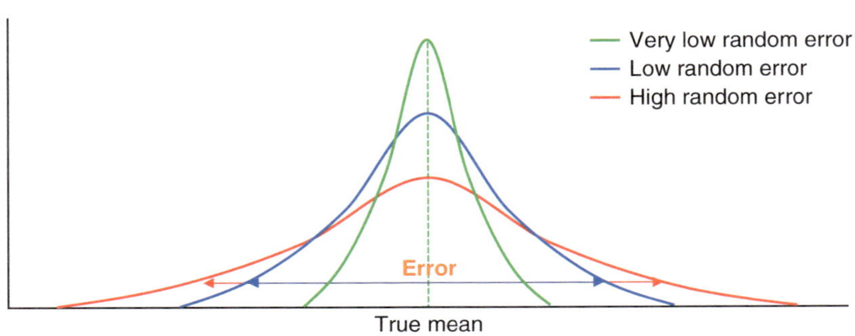

Fig. 9.3 Variation in results due to random error

3. Discuss the potential consequences of random error in epidemiological research for public health policy and practice. How can flawed data influence decision-making?

9.4 Systematic Error (Bias)

Description

Systematic error, also known as bias, is a *consistent* deviation from the true value that impacts the *accuracy* of results. It occurs when there are flaws in participant *selection* or data *collection* methods, resulting in observed findings that differ from the true values. As illustrated in Fig. 9.4, bias can either *overestimate* or *underestimate* effects and can arise at any stage of a study, from design to analysis. It is categorized into *selection* bias and *information* bias [7, 8].

Example for Selection Bias

In a study investigating the effectiveness of a new weight loss program, researchers recruit participants from a local gym. Since gym-goers are generally more health-conscious and likely to engage in regular physical activity, this sample may not represent the broader population, which includes individuals with varying levels of fitness and lifestyle choices. As a result, the findings may suggest that the weight loss program is more effective than it truly is for the general population, leading to an overestimation of its effectiveness due to the selection bias.

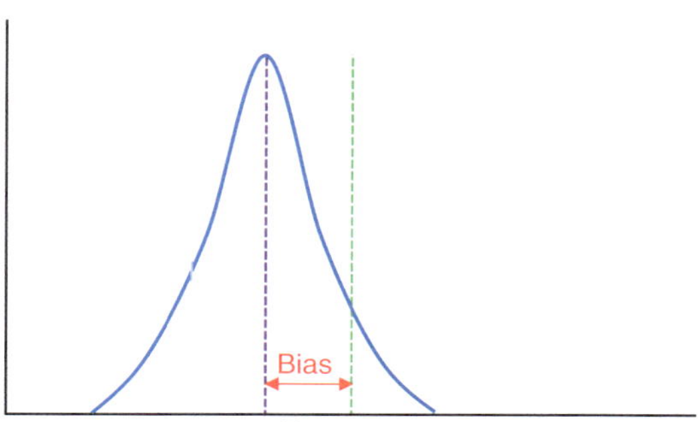

Fig. 9.4 Biased distribution due to systematic error

Example for Information Bias

In a study investigating the relationship between body mass index (BMI) and cardiovascular disease (CVD), researchers relied on self-reported weight and height from participants to calculate BMI. For instance, a participant who actually weighs 85 kg might report their weight as 80 kg due to social desirability bias, wanting to appear healthier. This misreporting leads to information bias, as the study may inaccurately associate a lower BMI with a reduced risk of CVD, ultimately distorting the findings and potentially influencing public health recommendations. To reduce such bias, researchers could use objective measurements instead of relying solely on self-reported data.

Conceptual Questions

1. Define systematic errors (also known as bias) in the context of epidemiological studies. What are some common sources of systematic errors, and how can they affect study outcomes?
2. Explain how systematic error can lead to either overestimation or underestimation of effects. What are the potential consequences of these inaccuracies for public health interventions and policy decisions?
3. How can researchers identify the presence of systematic error in their studies?

9.4.1 Selection Bias

Description

Selection bias occurs when the study participants are *not representative* of the target population. Errors in selecting study participants can lead to different probabilities of being included in the study sample resulting in a biased sample, as shown in Table 9.2. Consequently, an apparent association between exposure and outcome may be observed when, in reality, none exists [8, 85].

The red arrow in Table 9.2 indicates that exposed patients are more likely to be selected for inclusion in the study sample than their actual

Table 9.2 Selection bias: disproportionate representation in sample

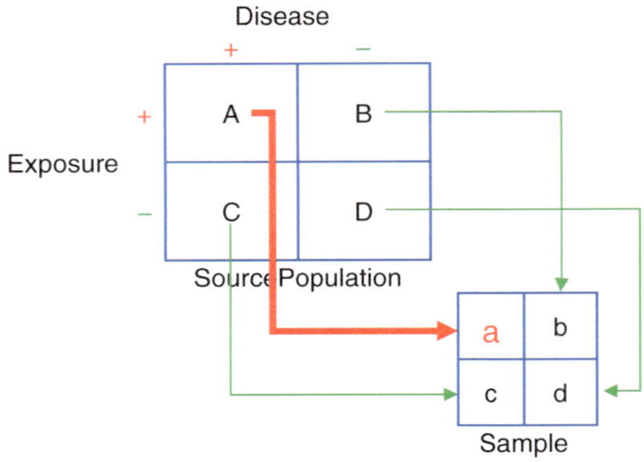

The remaining study population may no longer accurately represent the original sample, leading to biased estimates.

- Hospitalized patients: Studies conducted in hospital settings may overrepresent individuals with severe illnesses, potentially leading to an overestimation of the association between certain risk factors and the disease.
- Healthy worker effect: Studies conducted in occupational settings may underestimate the health risks associated with certain exposures because healthier individuals are more likely to be employed and included in the study population.

proportion in the source population. This means that the sampling method used in the study is biased toward including individuals who have been exposed to a specific risk factor. As a result, the sample may contain a higher percentage of exposed patients than what is representative of the general population. This overrepresentation can lead to an exaggerated perception of the relationship between the exposure and the disease of interest.

Examples for Selection Bias

- Enrollment of old cases: Studies that focus on prevalent (old) cases rather than incident (new) cases may overrepresent cases with longer disease duration and milder symptoms, potentially leading to an underestimation of disease severity.
- Nonresponse (refusal): When individuals refuse to participate in a study, the resulting sample may not be representative of the target population. Those who agree to participate may differ systematically from those who decline, potentially introducing bias into the study.
- Self-selection (volunteers): Studies that rely on volunteers may attract individuals with specific characteristics, such as a higher level of health consciousness or particular risk factors, which can lead to a biased sample.
- Differential losses to follow-up: Occur when participants drop out of a study at varying rates based on their exposure or disease status.

Conceptual Questions

1. Define selection bias in the context of epidemiological studies. How does it differ from other types of bias, such as information bias?
2. Discuss how selection bias affects the representativeness of a study sample compared to the target population. What are the potential consequences of having a biased sample on the study's findings?
3. Explain how focusing on prevalent cases rather than incident cases can lead to an underestimation of disease severity. What implications does this have for understanding the true burden of disease in the population?
4. How can nonresponse (refusal) introduce bias into a study? Discuss the characteristics that may differ between those who participate and those who decline and how this affects study outcomes.
5. Discuss the implications of self-selection in studies that rely on volunteers. How might the characteristics of volunteers skew the results compared to a randomly selected sample?
6. Explain how differential losses to follow-up can create selection bias. What factors might influence participants' decisions to drop out of a study, and how can this affect the validity of the study's conclusions?
7. How does conducting studies in hospital settings potentially overrepresent severe illnesses? Discuss how this might lead to an overestimation of the association between risk factors and diseases.

8. Define the healthy worker effect and discuss its implications for studies conducted in occupational settings. How can this bias lead to an underestimation of health risks associated with certain exposures?

9.4.2 Information Bias

Description

Information bias, also known as *misclassification*, occurs when there are inaccuracies in measuring exposure or outcome variables. Table 9.3 demonstrates how systematic measurement errors result in the misclassification of data [8, 85].

Table 9.3 illustrates the concept of information bias in epidemiological studies, emphasizing how errors in diagnosing exposure (in case-control studies) or outcomes (in cohort studies) can lead to the misclassification of participants, resulting in a sample that is not representative of the target population. The red arrow indicates misdiagnosis and subsequent misclassification of participants. The thick arrows represent a higher degree of misclassification, leading to a disproportionate sample compared to their actual proportions in the target population. This misrepresentation can result in biased estimations of the association between the exposure and the disease. Consequently, such overrepresentation may distort the perceived strength of the relationship, potentially leading to misleading conclusions about the exposure's impact on health outcomes.

Examples for Information Bias

- Recall bias: Also known as *rumination* bias, this occurs when participants with a particular disease or outcome have better recall of past exposures compared to those without the disease.
- Imperfect sensitivity: Occurs when a diagnostic test fails to identify individuals with the disease, resulting in false negatives. For instance, a screening test with low sensitivity may miss cases, leading to an underestimation of disease prevalence.
- Imperfect specificity: Occurs when a diagnostic test incorrectly identifies individuals without the disease as having the disease, resulting in false positives. A test with low specificity may overestimate the disease prevalence.

Conceptual Questions

1. Define information bias (misclassification) in the context of epidemiological studies. How does it differ from selection bias, and what are its key characteristics?
2. Discuss how information bias affects the accuracy of exposure and outcome measurements in studies. What are the potential consequences of misclassification on the validity of research findings?
3. Explain how recall bias can occur in case-control studies. Why might individuals with a particular disease have better recall of past exposures compared to those without the disease? What implications does this have for the study's findings?
4. Discuss the concept of imperfect sensitivity in diagnostic tests. How can false negatives lead to an underestimation of disease prevalence, and what are the potential consequences for public health?

Table 9.3 Information bias: impact of misclassification on exposure and outcome in case-control and cohort studies

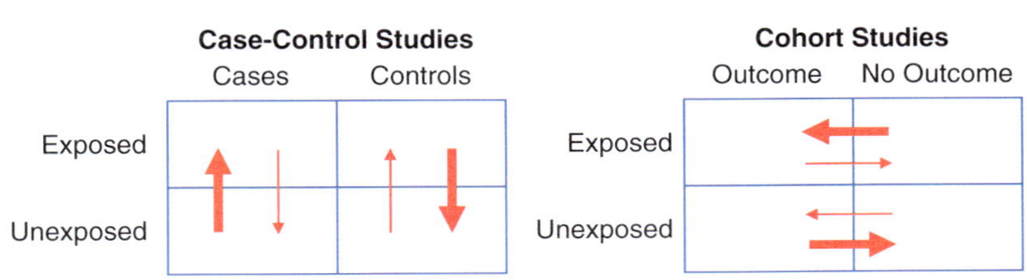

5. Define imperfect specificity and explain how it can result in false positives. What impact does this have on the perceived prevalence of a disease in a population?
6. How can information bias lead to incorrect conclusions about the relationship between exposure and outcome?

9.5 Confounding

Description

Confounding occurs when a third variable, known as a confounder, is associated with both the exposure and the outcome, distorting the true relationship between them. A confounder is a factor that is causally related to the outcome and either causally or noncausally related to the exposure; however, it is not an intermediate step in the causal pathway between the exposure and outcome [2, 7, 8], as illustrated in Fig. 9.5.

Essentially, confounding can distort the observed relationship, making it appear stronger, weaker, induced, eliminated, or even reversed [8]. When a confounding effect strengthens the relationship between exposure and outcome, it is referred to as a *positive* confounder. Conversely, if it weakens the relationship, it is considered a *negative* confounder. If the confounder reverses the relationship—transforming a protective association into a risk association or vice versa—it is classified as a *qualitative* confounder. Positive and negative confounders, on the other hand, are categorized as *quantitative* confounders because they alter the strength of the relationship without reversing its direction.

Examples 1: Cataract and Stroke

A hypothetical study aims to investigate the relationship between cataract and stroke. Age is considered a confounding factor because it is causally linked to both conditions. As depicted in Fig. 9.6, older individuals are more likely to experience both cataracts and strokes.

In this context, age serves as a confounding variable in the relationship between cataracts and stroke. Both conditions are more prevalent among older individuals, meaning that as people age, their risk of developing cataracts and experiencing strokes increases. Consequently, age can influence the likelihood of having either condition.

The figure suggests that cataracts do not have a direct causal effect on stroke. Instead, the observed association between cataracts and stroke may be misleading because of the influence of age. When age is taken into account, the apparent link between cataracts and stroke may diminish or disappear, indicating that it is age, rather than cataracts, that is driving the association.

When studying the relationship between cataracts and stroke, it is essential to control for age to avoid confounding. If researchers fail to account for age, they may incorrectly conclude that cataracts increase the risk of stroke, when, in fact, it is the aging process that contributes to both conditions.

Examples 2: Coffee Consumption and Coronary Heart Disease (CHD)

A study aims to explore the association between coffee consumption and CHD. Smoking is a con-

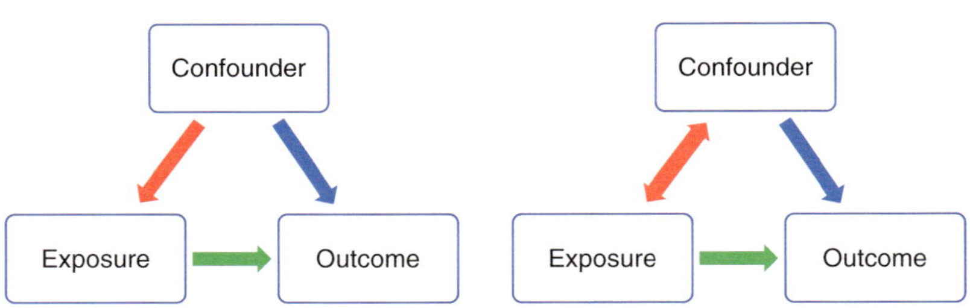

Fig. 9.5 The relationship between exposure, outcome, and confounding variable. Unidirectional arrows indicate causal relationships, while bidirectional arrows represent noncausal relationships

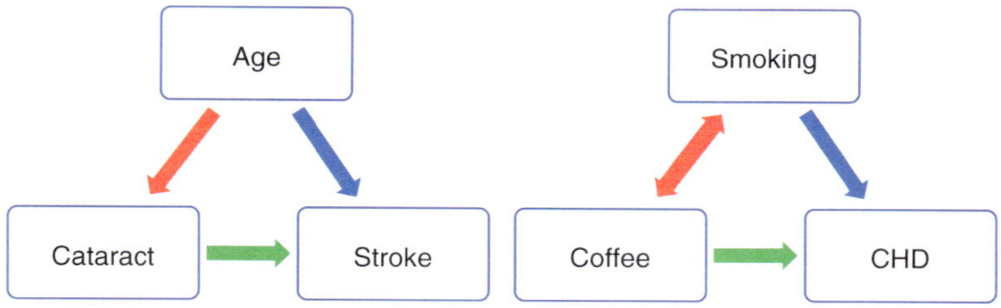

Fig. 9.6 Examples of confounding: age as a confounder in cataract and stroke; smoking as a confounder in coffee consumption and coronary heart disease (CHD)

founding variable because it is a known risk factor for CHD and may also be associated with coffee consumption habits. As illustrated in Fig. 9.6, individuals who smoke are more likely to have both CHD and higher rates of coffee consumption.

In this context, smoking acts as a confounding variable in the relationship between coffee consumption and CHD. It significantly increases the likelihood of developing heart disease, while research indicates that smokers tend to consume more coffee than nonsmokers. This creates a scenario where smoking influences both coffee consumption and the risk of CHD.

The figure suggests that the relationship between coffee consumption and CHD may not be direct. Instead, the observed association could largely be attributed to smoking. If researchers do not account for smoking, they might mistakenly conclude that coffee consumption directly increases the risk of CHD, when, in reality, it is smoking that drives both the higher coffee consumption and the increased risk of heart disease.

When studying the relationship between coffee consumption and CHD, it is essential to control for smoking to avoid confounding. Failing to do so could lead to erroneous interpretations, suggesting that coffee itself poses a risk for CHD, while the underlying risk factor is actually smoking.

Examples 3: Having a Lighter and Lung Cancer

In this example, we examine a hypothetical case-control study where the observed association between the exposure and the outcome is entirely attributable to the confounding effect. Specifically, the study investigates the relationship between having a lighter (exposure) and lung cancer (outcome), with smoking acting as the confounding variable, as illustrated in Fig. 9.7.

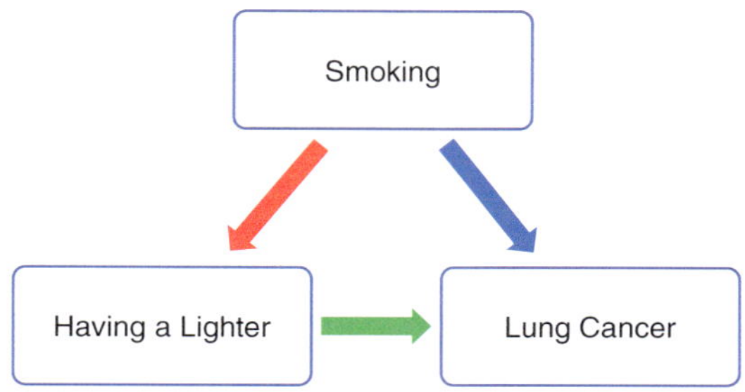

Fig. 9.7 Examples of confounding: the role of smoking as a confounder in the relationship between having a lighter and lung cancer

As shown in Table 9.4, the crude odds ratio (OR) of 8.8 suggests that individuals who possess a lighter are approximately 8.8 times more likely to develop lung cancer compared to those who do not possess a lighter. However, this association may be misleading due to the potential confounding effect of smoking. Lighters are commonly used by smokers, and smoking is a well-established risk factor for lung cancer. Therefore, the elevated odds ratio could reflect the underlying influence of smoking rather than a direct causal relationship between lighter possession and lung cancer.

The association between having a lighter and lung cancer, when analyzed separately for smokers and nonsmokers, is presented in Table 9.5. In both groups, the odds ratio of 1.0 indicates that there is no significant association between having a lighter and lung cancer. This suggests that, when analyzed separately, the presence of a lighter does not increase the risk of lung cancer in either group. The absence of an association in both subgroups underscores the importance of considering smoking as a confounding factor.

Table 9.4 Association between having a lighter and lung cancer, failing to consider smoking as a confounding factor

Exposure	Cases (Lung Cancer)	Controls (No Lung Cancer)	Odds Ratio
Having a lighter	820	340	$OR = \frac{820 \times 660}{340 \times 180} = 8.8$
Not having a lighter	180	660	
Total	1000	1000	

Table 9.5 Association between having a lighter and lung cancer in smokers and nonsmokers

	Exposure	Cases	Controls	Odds Ratio
Smokers	Having a lighter	810	270	$OR = \frac{810 \times 30}{270 \times 90} = 1.0$
	Not having a lighter	90	30	
	Total	900	300	
Nonsmokers	Having a lighter	10	70	$OR = \frac{10 \times 630}{70 \times 90} = 1.0$
	Not having a lighter	90	630	
	Total	100	700	

As illustrated above, one effective approach to identify a confounding factor is through stratification based on the confounding variable, as shown in Table 9.5. When a confounding effect is present, the associations observed across the strata of the potentially confounding variable are of *similar* magnitude (e.g., OR = 1.0), yet they *differ* significantly from the crude estimate (e.g., OR = 8.8). In the example provided, the entire association between lighter use and lung cancer can be attributed to the confounding effect of smoking, which is causally related to lung cancer and also associated with lighter use.

Another approach to assess the confounding effect of smoking is to calculate the Mantel-Haenszel odds ratio (OR_{MH}) and compare it with the crude OR. The OR_{MH} represents a weighted average of the OR calculated separately for smokers and nonsmokers, allowing for adjustment of the association for the potential confounding factor. A significant difference between the OR_{MH} and the crude OR indicates the presence of a confounding factor:

$$OR_{MH} = \frac{\sum_{i=1}^{k} \frac{a_i d_i}{n_i}}{\sum_{i=1}^{k} \frac{b_i c_i}{n_i}} = \frac{\frac{810 \times 30}{1200} + \frac{10 \times 630}{800}}{\frac{270 \times 90}{1200} + \frac{70 \times 90}{800}} = 1.0$$

In the present analysis, the adjusted odds ratio (OR_{MH}) was calculated and found to be equal to 1.0. This result suggests that the observed association between possession of a lighter and lung cancer is entirely attributable to confounding by smoking. Specifically, after accounting for smoking status, no significant association remains between having a lighter and the risk of lung cancer. These findings underscore the importance of controlling for confounding variables to ensure accurate interpretation of associations in epidemiological studies.

Conceptual Questions

1. Define confounding in the context of epidemiological studies. How does it differ from bias, and what role does a confounder play in distorting the relationship between exposure and outcome?

2. Describe the characteristics of a confounder. What criteria must a variable meet to be considered a confounder in a study?
3. How can confounding distort the observed relationship between exposure and outcome? Provide examples of how confounding can make an association appear stronger, weaker, induced, eliminated, or even reversed.
4. What methods can researchers employ to control for confounding in their studies? Discuss techniques such as randomization, restriction, matching, and statistical adjustment (e.g., multivariable regression).
5. What are the potential consequences of failing to account for confounding in epidemiological research? Discuss how this failure can result in misleading conclusions and affect public health recommendations.

9.6 Interaction

Description

Interaction, also known as *effect modification*, occurs when two or more risk factors influence each other's effects on the occurrence or intensity of a specific outcome, as illustrated in Fig. 9.8. In simpler terms, when interaction is present, the combined impact of the factors on an outcome is either greater or lesser than the effect of each factor alone. There are two types of interactions:

Synergistic (Positive) Interaction

The combined effect of two factors is *greater* than the sum of their individual effects, amplifying the outcome, as illustrated in Fig. 9.9.

Example

Individuals who smoke have a certain risk of developing lung cancer, and those exposed to asbestos also face a risk. However, when a person is both a smoker and has been exposed to asbestos, their risk of lung cancer is significantly higher than the sum of the risks from each exposure alone. This illustrates how the combination of smoking and asbestos exposure amplifies the overall health risk, highlighting the importance of understanding how different factors can interact to influence health outcomes.

Antagonistic (Negative) Interaction

The combined effect of two factors is *less* than the sum of their individual effects, reducing the impact of one or both factors, as illustrated in Fig. 9.9.

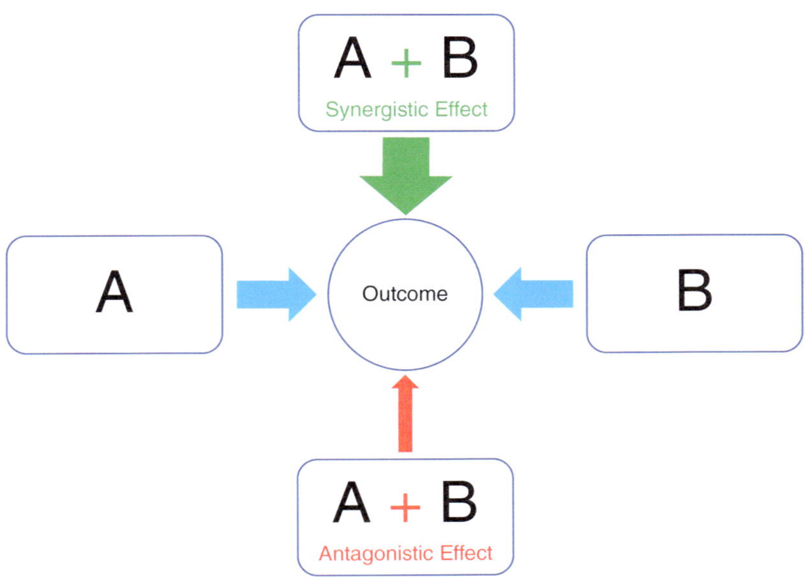

Fig. 9.8 Interactive effects of factors A and B on outcome. The thickness of the arrows indicates the magnitude of the effect, with thicker arrows representing larger effects and thinner arrows representing smaller effects

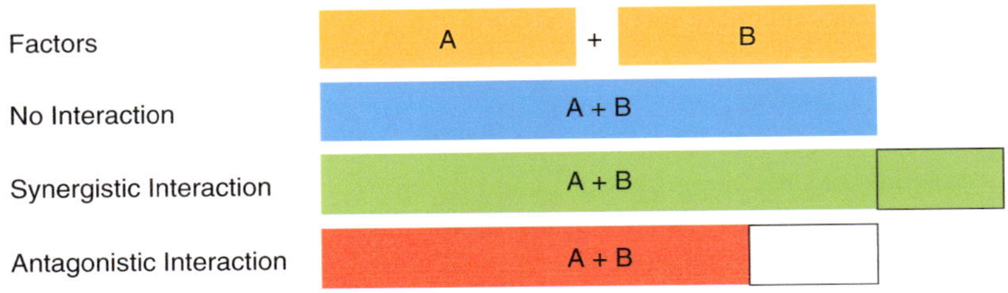

Fig. 9.9 Joint and independent effects of factors A and B

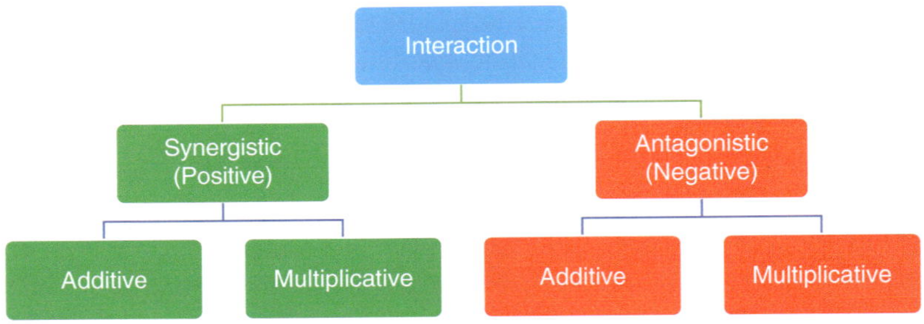

Fig. 9.10 Models of interaction: additive vs. multiplicative

Example
Obesity is a well-established risk factor for cardiovascular disease (CVD). Excess body weight can lead to increased blood pressure, elevated cholesterol levels, and insulin resistance, all of which contribute to the development of CVD. Conversely, regular physical activity is known to have protective effects against CVD. It helps maintain a healthy weight, lowers blood pressure, improves lipid profiles, and enhances insulin sensitivity.

For individuals who are obese, engaging in regular physical activity can significantly mitigate the negative health impacts associated with excess weight. For example, an obese person who exercises regularly may have a lower risk of developing CVD compared to an obese individual who is sedentary. Thus, while obesity is a risk factor for cardiovascular disease, regular physical activity can counteract some of the adverse effects of obesity, illustrating a complex interaction between these two risk factors.

However, the effectiveness of physical activity in reducing CVD risk may also be influenced by the degree of obesity. Individuals with severe obesity may face greater challenges in achieving the same cardiovascular benefits from physical activity as those with a lower body weight. Factors such as joint pain, reduced mobility, and other obesity-related health issues can limit the intensity and duration of physical activity, potentially diminishing its protective effects.

This example highlights the interaction between these two factors, where physical activity can diminish or negate the harmful effects of obesity on health outcomes, while obesity can similarly reduce the cardiovascular benefits gained from physical activity.

Approaches to Evaluating Interaction Effects
A crucial aspect of evaluating interaction is deciding how to measure their effect. As illustrated in Fig. 9.10, this can be accomplished using either an additive model (such as risk difference or mean difference) or a multiplicative model (such as risk ratio, rate ratio, hazard ratio, or odds ratio).

Two approaches can be used to evaluate interactions:

Homogeneity/Heterogeneity Approach
This approach assesses whether the effect of an independent variable on the dependent variable remains consistent across different levels of another independent variable. If the effect is consistent (homogeneous) across all levels of the other independent variable, it indicates the absence of an interaction effect. Conversely, if the effect varies

(heterogeneous) across these levels, it suggests the presence of an interaction effect. By examining homogeneity, researchers can determine whether the relationship between the independent and dependent variables is stable or if it significantly changes depending on the levels of the interacting variable. This approach provides valuable insights into the potential moderating role of the interacting variable in the observed relationship.

Observed/Expected Approach

This approach involves comparing the observed interaction effect to the expected interaction effect under the null hypothesis of no interaction. If the observed and expected effects are similar, this indicates the absence of an interaction effect. Conversely, if the observed and expected effects differ significantly, it suggests the presence of an interaction effect. By evaluating discrepancies between the observed outcomes and those anticipated under the null hypothesis, researchers can gain valuable insights into the nature, magnitude, and significance of the interaction.

The following sections will provide a detailed discussion of these approaches, highlighting their methodologies, applications, and implications for understanding interaction effects in research.

Homogeneity/Heterogeneity Approach

When using the homogeneity/heterogeneity approach, if there is no interaction, the effect measure remains consistent across strata, indicating *homogeneity*. However, if there is an interaction, the effect measure will vary across strata, indicating *heterogeneity*.

Table 9.6 evaluates various scenarios of *additive* interaction using the homogeneity/heterogeneity approach. In the absence of additive interaction, the risk difference for factor B remains constant regardless of whether factor A is present or absent. When *synergistic* additive interaction is present, the risk difference for factor B is higher when factor A is present compared to when it is absent. Conversely, in cases of *antagonistic* additive interaction, the risk difference for factor B is lower when factor A is present.

Table 9.6 Additive interaction—a hypothetical example

	A	B	Incidence Risk (per1000)	Risk Difference
Absence of Additive Interaction (No Interaction)	No	No	20.0	Ref.
		Yes	40.0	20.0
	Yes	No	50.0	Ref.
		Yes	70.0	20.0

	A	B	Incidence Risk (per 1000)	Risk Difference
Presence of Additive Interaction (Synergistic)	No	No	20.0	Ref.
		Yes	40.0	20.0
	Yes	No	50.0	Ref.
		Yes	90.0	40.0

	A	B	Incidence Risk (per 1000)	Risk Difference
Presence of Additive Interaction (Antagonistic)	No	No	20.0	Ref.
		Yes	40.0	20.0
	Yes	No	50.0	Ref.
		Yes	60.0	10.0

Table 9.7 Multiplicative interaction—a hypothetical example

Scenario	A	B	Incidence Risk (per 1000)	Risk Ratio
Absence of Multiplicative Interaction (No Interaction)	No	No	20.0	Ref.
		Yes	40.0	2.0
	Yes	No	30.0	Ref.
		Yes	60.0	2.0
Presence of Multiplicative Interaction (Synergistic)	No	No	20.0	Ref.
		Yes	40.0	2.0
	Yes	No	30.0	Ref.
		Yes	90.0	3.0
Presence of Multiplicative Interaction (Antagonistic)	No	No	20.0	Ref.
		Yes	40.0	2.0
	Yes	No	50.0	Ref.
		Yes	80.0	1.6

Table 9.7 evaluates various scenarios of *multiplicative* interaction using the homogeneity/heterogeneity approach. When there is no multiplicative interaction, the risk ratio for factor B remains constant regardless of whether factor A is present or absent. However, in the presence of *synergistic* multiplicative interaction, the risk ratio for factor B is higher when factor A is present compared to when it is absent. Conversely, in cases of *antagonistic* multiplicative interaction, the risk ratio for factor B is lower when factor A is present.

Observed/Expected Approach

When using the observed/expected approach, the absence of interaction is characterized by identical joint observed and expected effects. Conversely, if interaction is present, these joint effects will differ.

Table 9.8 evaluates various scenarios of *additive* interaction using the observed/expected approach. When there is no additive interaction, the joint observed and expected risk differences for factors A and B are equal. However, if there is *synergistic* additive interaction, the joint *observed* risk difference for factors A and B is greater than the joint

Table 9.8 A hypothetical example: additive interaction using observed/expected approach

Absence of Additive Interaction (No Interaction)

	Incidence Risk (per 1000) B −	Incidence Risk (per 1000) B +		Risk Difference B −	Risk Difference B +
A −	20.0	40.0	A −	0.0	20.0
A +	50.0	70.0	A +	30.0	50.0

Joint Expected Risk Difference = 20.0 + 30.0 = 50.0 / 1000
Joint Observed Risk Difference = 50.0 / 1000
Joint Observed Risk Difference = Joint Expected Risk Difference
⇨ No Additive Interaction

Presence of Additive Interaction (Synergistic)

	Incidence Risk (per 1000) B −	Incidence Risk (per 1000) B +		Risk Difference B −	Risk Difference B +
A −	20.0	40.0	A −	0.0	20.0
A +	50.0	90.0	A +	30.0	70.0

Joint Expected Risk Difference = 20.0 + 30.0 = 50.0 / 1000
Joint Observed Risk Difference = 70.0 / 1000
Joint Observed Risk Difference > Joint Expected Risk Difference
⇨ SynergisticInteraction

Presence of Additive Interaction (Antagonistic)

	Incidence Risk (per 1000) B −	Incidence Risk (per 1000) B +		Risk Difference B −	Risk Difference B +
A −	20.0	40.0	A −	0.0	20.0
A +	50.0	60.0	A +	30.0	40.0

Joint Expected Risk Difference = 20.0 + 30.0 = 50.0 / 1000
Joint Observed Risk Difference = 40.0 / 1000
Joint Observed Risk Difference < Joint Expected Risk Difference
⇨ AntagonisticInteraction

expected risk difference. Conversely, *antagonistic* additive interaction results in a smaller joint *observed* risk difference compared to the joint *expected* risk difference for factors A and B.

Table 9.9 evaluates various scenarios of *multiplicative* interaction using the observed/expected approach. When there is no multiplicative interaction, the joint observed and expected risk ratios for factors A and B are equal. If there is a *synergistic* multiplicative interaction, the joint *observed* risk ratio for factors A and B is higher than the joint *expected* risk ratio. Conversely, in the case of an *antagonistic* multiplicative interaction, the joint *observed* risk ratio for factors A and B will be lower than the joint *expected* risk ratio.

Table 9.9 A hypothetical example: multiplicative interaction using observed/expected approach

Absence of Multiplicative Interaction (No Interaction)

Incidence Risk (per 1000)

		B -	B +
A	-	20.0	40.0
A	+	30.0	60.0

Risk Ratio

		B -	B +
A	-	1.0	2.0
A	+	1.5	3.0

Joint Expected Risk Ratio = 2.0 ×+ 1.5 = **3.0**
Joint Observed Risk Radio = **3.0**
Joint Observed Risk Radio = Joint Expected Risk Ratio ⇨ No Multiplicative Interaction

Presence of Multiplicative Interaction (Synergistic)

Incidence Risk (per 1000)

		B -	B +
A	-	20.0	40.0
A	+	30.0	90.0

Risk Ratio

		B -	B +
A	-	1.0	2.0
A	+	1.5	4.5

Joint Expected Risk Ratio = 2.0 × 1.5 = **3.0**
Joint Observed Risk Radio = **4.5**
Joint Observed Risk Radio > Joint Expected Risk Ratio ⇨ Synergistic Interaction

Presence of Multiplicative Interaction (Antagonistic)

Incidence Risk (per 1000)

		B -	B +
A	-	20.0	40.0
A	+	50.0	80.0

Risk Ratio

	B -	B +
	1.0	2.0
	2.5	4.0

Joint Expected Risk Ratio = 2.0 × 2.5 = **5.0**
Joint Observed Risk Radio = **4.0**
Joint Observed Risk Radio < Joint Expected Risk Ratio ⇨ Antagonistic Interaction

Conceptual Questions

1. Define interaction (effect modification) in the context of epidemiological studies. How does interaction differ from confounding, and what role does it play in understanding the relationship between exposure and outcome?
2. Describe the two types of interactions: synergistic (positive) interaction and antagonistic (negative) interaction. Provide examples of each type and discuss how they influence the overall effect on an outcome.
3. Discuss the difference between additive and multiplicative models of interaction. How do these models help researchers measure the combined effects of multiple factors on an outcome?
4. Explain the homogeneity/heterogeneity approach to assessing interaction. How can researchers determine whether the effect of one independent variable on the dependent variable is consistent across different levels of another variable?
5. Describe the observed/expected approach to evaluating interactions. How can this method help researchers identify the presence of interaction between factors?
6. What statistical techniques can be employed to assess and model interaction in epidemiological data? Discuss methods such as interaction terms in regression analysis and how they can be interpreted.

10 Protocol Deviation in Randomized Controlled Trials

Contents

10.1 Protocol Deviation in RCTs: Analysis and Approaches

Description
A protocol deviation refers to any departure from the study procedures or treatment plans specified in the approved protocol. In simpler terms, it occurs when an aspect of a clinical trial does not adhere to the original plan [2, 49]. Protocol deviations can happen for various reasons, including:

- Refusing the assigned treatment
- Receiving the wrong treatment
- Misunderstandings of instructions
- Reluctance to follow a strict schedule
- Difficulties in adhering to the regimen
- Unforeseen medical conditions

As illustrated in Fig. 10.1, a hypothetical randomized controlled trial (RCT) randomly assigned participants to receive either medical or surgical treatment. However, some patients in both groups deviated from the assigned treatment by refusing it and receiving alternative treatment. Several approaches have been suggested to address this protocol deviation.

10.1.1 Intention-to-Treat (ITT) Analysis

This approach analyzes all participants as if they followed their assigned treatment, regardless of actual adherence. This approach preserves the randomization process and provides a more conservative estimate of the treatment effect in the real world.

10.1.2 Per-Protocol Analysis

This approach analyzes only participants who strictly adhered to their assigned treatment. This approach provides a more ideal estimate of the treatment effect but may not be representative of the real-world population.

10.1.3 As-Treated Analysis

This approach analyzes participants based on the treatment they actually received. This approach provides an estimate of the treatment effect under

J. Poorolajal, *Illustrated Epidemiology*, https://doi.org/10.1007/978-981-96-9566-9_10

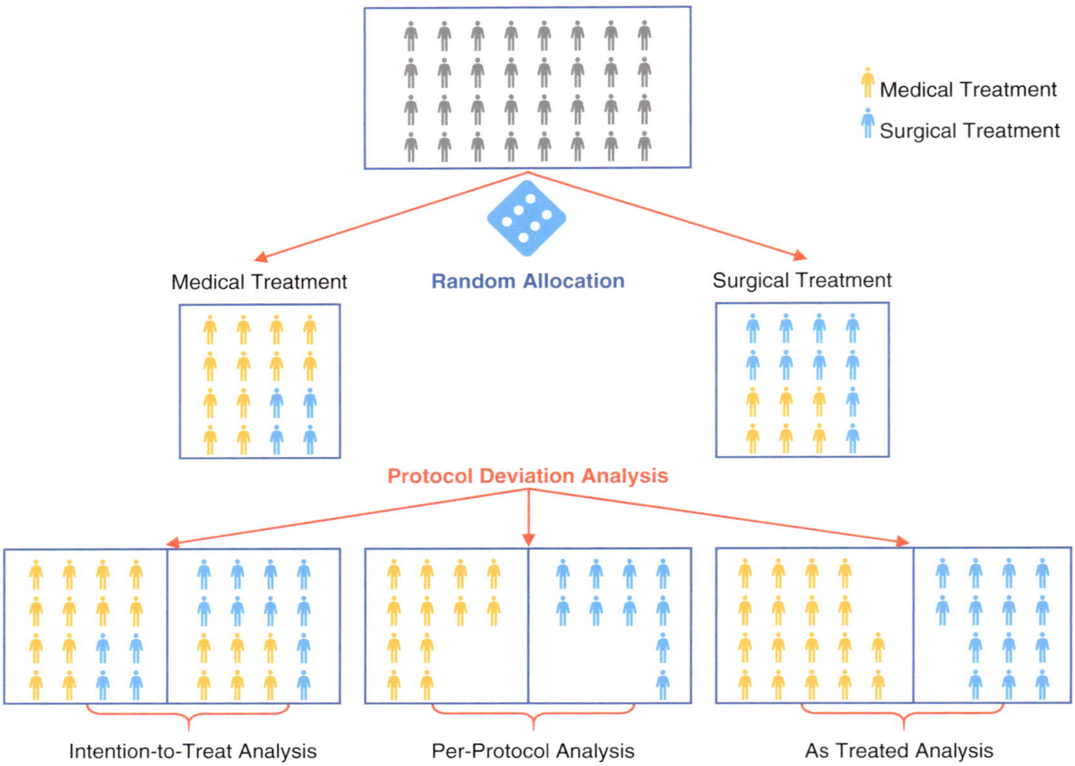

Fig. 10.1 Randomized controlled trial (RCT) with treatment deviations: analysis strategies

Fig. 10.2 A hypothetical randomized controlled trial with protocol deviations

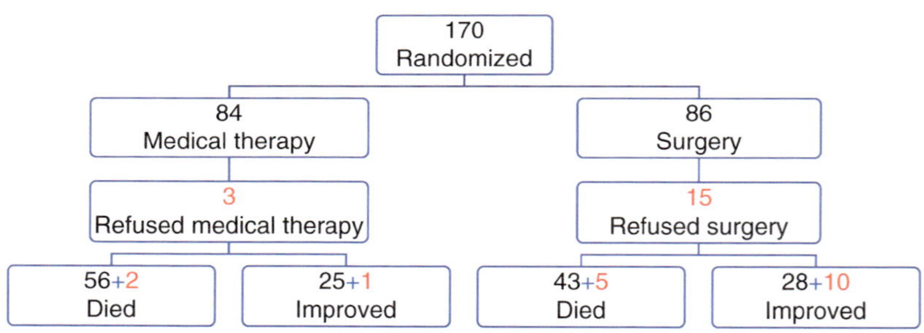

real-world conditions but may not be suitable for causal inference due to *self-selection bias*.

Example 1
Figure 10.2 illustrates the results of a hypothetical randomized clinical trial (RCT) that enrolled 170 patients. These patients were randomly assigned to either medical therapy or surgery. Out of the participants, 86 were assigned to surgery and 84 to medical therapy. Eighteen patients refused their assigned treatments, with 15 from the surgical group opting for medical therapy and three from the medical therapy group choosing surgery. The results of this trial are summarized in Table 10.1. The trial outcome, improvement, was analyzed using three approaches: intention-to-treat, per-protocol, and as-treated analysis, with medical therapy as the reference group.

Intention-to-Treat (ITT) Analysis
The fundamental principle in ITT analysis is to analyze all participants based on their original

Table 10.1 A hypothetical randomized controlled trial with protocol deviations

Randomized group	Randomized to medical therapy, $n = 84$		Randomized to surgery, $n = 86$	
Outcome	Took medical therapy	Took surgery	Took surgery	Took medical therapy
Improved	25	1	28	10
Not improved	56	2	43	5
Total	81	3	71	15

treatment assignment, regardless of whether they actually completed the treatment or not.

Advantages
- Preserves randomization
- Reflects *real-world* effectiveness
- Provides a conservative estimate of treatment effect

Disadvantages
- Can underestimate the true treatment effect if many patients drop out or do not adhere to the treatment

Formula

$$\text{Risk ratio} = \frac{38/86}{26/84} = 1.43$$

The results of this RCT suggest that based on an "intention-to-treat analysis," patients who underwent surgery were 1.43 times more likely to show improvement compared to those who received medical therapy.

Per-Protocol Analysis
This analysis includes only participants who strictly adhered to the treatment plan.

Advantages
- Provides an estimate of the treatment effect under *ideal* conditions

Disadvantages
- May not reflect real-world effectiveness
- Risk of selection bias

Formula

$$\text{Risk ratio} = \frac{28/71}{25/81} = 1.28$$

The results of this RCT suggest that based on a "per-protocol analysis," patients who underwent surgery were 1.28 times more likely to improve compared to those who received medical therapy.

As-Treated Analysis
This analysis evaluates participants based on the treatment they actually received, regardless of their assigned group.

Advantages
- May provide a more realistic estimate of treatment effect

Disadvantages
- Can compromise randomization
- Risk of self-selection bias
- May be confounded by baseline differences

Formula

$$\text{Risk ratio} = \frac{29/74}{35/96} = 1.07$$

The results of this RCT suggest that based on an "as-treated analysis," patients who underwent surgery were 1.07 times more likely to improve compared to those who received medical therapy.

Example 2
As illustrated in Fig. 10.3, the conservative management versus tonsillectomy in adults with recurrent acute tonsillitis in the UK (NATTINA) trial aimed to assess the clinical effectiveness and cost-effectiveness of these two approaches. A total of 453 eligible participants were randomly assigned to two groups: 233 to the immediate tonsillectomy group and 220 to the conservative management group. In the immediate tonsillectomy group, after excluding nine participants who did not have primary outcome data, 224 were included in the primary intention-to-treat (ITT) analysis, although 61 did not receive the

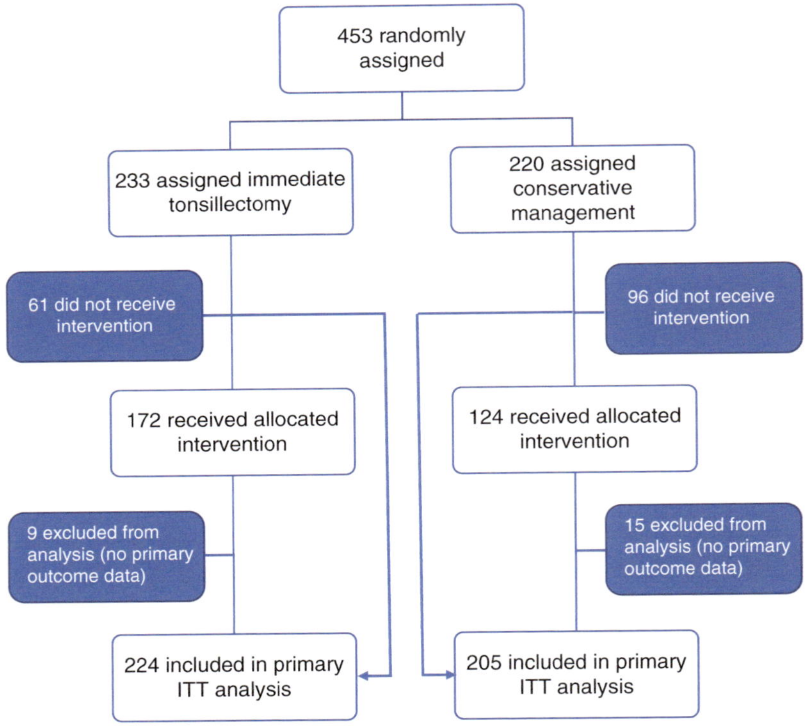

Fig. 10.3 Randomized controlled trial (RCT) with treatment deviations analyzed using intention-to-treat (ITT) approach

allocated intervention. In the conservative management group, after excluding 15 participants without primary outcome data, 205 were included in the primary ITT analysis, despite 96 not receiving the allocated intervention [86].

To analyze the results of the same study using the per-protocol method, we will focus exclusively on patients who adhered to the assigned treatment protocols. In the immediate tonsillectomy group, 172 patients received the intervention; after excluding 9 patients without available primary outcome data, 163 patients will be included in the analysis. In the conservative management group, 124 patients received the intervention; after excluding 15 patients without available primary outcome data, 109 patients will be included in the analysis. This approach will enable us to evaluate the outcomes based on adherence to the assigned treatments.

Conceptual Questions

1. Define protocol deviation in the context of randomized controlled trials. What are some common reasons for protocol deviations to occur in clinical research?
2. Discuss how protocol deviations can affect the validity and reliability of RCT results. What implications do these deviations have for the interpretation of treatment effects?
3. Explain the rationale behind using ITT analysis in RCTs. What are the advantages and disadvantages of this approach? How does it help preserve the integrity of randomization?
4. What is the purpose of conducting a per-protocol analysis? Discuss the advantages and disadvantages of this approach.
5. Describe the as-treated analysis approach. How does this method evaluate participants, and what are the potential biases associated with it? Why might this analysis be less suitable for causal inference?
6. Discuss the potential consequences of high rates of nonadherence to assigned treatments in RCTs. How might this affect the overall conclusions drawn from the study?

Statistical Concepts in Epidemiology

11

Contents

11.1 The Normal Curve

Description

A normal curve, commonly referred to as a *bell curve*, is a symmetrical probability distribution that is extensively utilized in statistics. It represents a dataset where most values cluster around the mean, with progressively fewer values occurring at the extremes, as illustrated in Fig. 11.1 [87]. The normal distribution is defined mathematically by its mean (μ) and standard deviation (σ), which dictate the center and spread of the curve, respectively.

Properties of a Normal Curve

- Symmetry: The curve is perfectly symmetrical around the mean, meaning that the left and right halves of the curve are mirror images of each other.
- Bell-shaped: The curve exhibits a distinctive bell-like shape, which is characteristic of many natural phenomena.
- Mean, median, and mode: In a normal distribution, the mean, median, and mode are all equal, providing a single central tendency measure.
- Standard deviation: The spread of the data is characterized by the standard deviation (σ). A smaller standard deviation indicates that the data points are closer to the mean, while a larger standard deviation signifies greater dispersion.
- Area under the curve: The total area under the curve is equal to one, representing the entirety of the probability distribution. This property allows for the calculation of probabilities associated with specific ranges of values.
- Empirical rule: Approximately 68% of the data falls within one standard deviation of the mean, 95% within two standard deviations, and 99.7% within three standard deviations. This rule is essential for understanding the distribution of data in various fields.

Importance of the Normal Curve

The normal curve is fundamental in statistics due to its properties and the central limit theorem, which states that the distribution of sample means will tend to be normal, regardless of the shape of the population distribution, provided the sample size is sufficiently large. This theorem underpins many statistical methods and hypothesis testing,

J. Poorolajal, *Illustrated Epidemiology*, https://doi.org/10.1007/978-981-96-9566-9_11

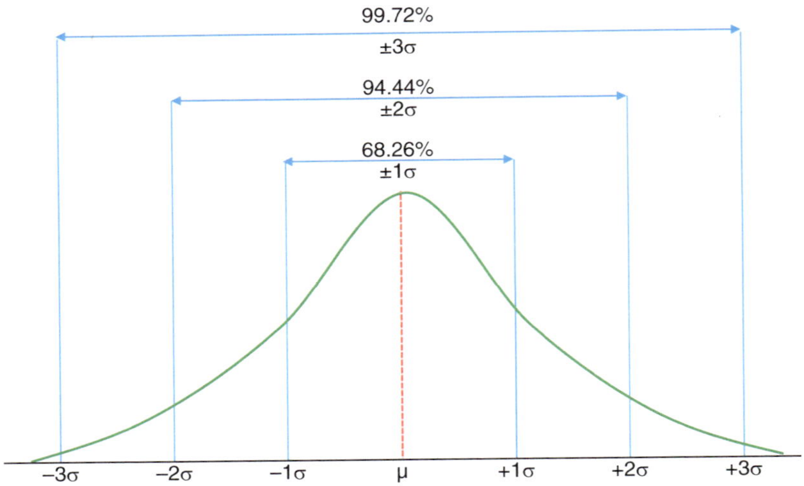

Fig. 11.1 Normal distribution: area under the curve by standard deviation

making the normal distribution a cornerstone of inferential statistics.

Applications of the Normal Curve in Epidemiology

In the field of epidemiology, the normal distribution plays a critical role in analyzing health-related data. Here are several key applications:

- Modeling population health data: Epidemiologists frequently utilize the normal curve to model the distribution of continuous health-related variables, such as blood pressure, cholesterol levels, and body mass index (BMI) within a population. By understanding the normal distribution of these variables, researchers can effectively describe population health metrics, identify outliers, and establish normative values for clinical assessments.
- Statistical inference: Many statistical tests used in epidemiology, such as t-tests and ANOVA, assume that the data follows a normal distribution. This assumption allows researchers to draw conclusions about population parameters based on sample data, facilitating the comparison of different groups or treatment effects.
- Data interpretation and visualization: The normal curve aids epidemiologists in understanding the distribution of health outcomes and risk factors within a population. By comparing observed data to the expected distribution, researchers can identify outliers or unusual patterns that may require further investigation.

Conceptual Questions

1. What is a normal curve, and why is it commonly referred to as a bell curve? Describe its key characteristics.
2. Explain the significance of symmetry in a normal distribution. How does this property affect the interpretation of data?
3. In a normal distribution, how are the mean, median, and mode related? Why is this relationship important for understanding the data?
4. How does the standard deviation (σ) influence the shape of the normal curve? Provide an example to illustrate your point.
5. Why is the total area under the normal curve equal to 1? How does this property facilitate probability calculations?
6. Describe the empirical rule. How can this rule be applied in real-world scenarios, particularly in health data analysis?
7. How do epidemiologists use the normal curve to model population health data? Provide specific examples of health-related variables that might be analyzed.

11.2 Standard Deviation Versus Standard Error

Standard Deviation (SD)

- Definition: The standard deviation measures the amount of *variation* or dispersion of *individual data* points around the population or sample mean, indicating how much variation exits among individuals [87].
- Importance: SD is crucial for *descriptive* statistics to describe the *variability* of data within a population. A smaller SD indicates that the data points are closely clustered around the mean, while a larger SD suggests greater variability.
- Application: SD is used in descriptive statistics to summarize data, allowing researchers to understand the distribution and variability of individual observations.

Standard Error (SE)

- Definition: The standard error measures the *variability* of *sample means* around the true population mean, informing us how much we can expect sample means to differ from the true population mean [87]. It is calculated as the standard deviation divided by the square root of the sample size ($SE = SD / \sqrt{n}$).
- Importance: SE is essential for *inferential* statistics, as it provides insight into the reliability and *precision* of sample estimates. A smaller SE indicates a more precise estimate of the population mean.
- Application: SE is commonly used in hypothesis testing and confidence interval estimation, helping researchers assess the uncertainty of sample statistics when making inferences about the population.

Example

Figure 11.2 displays a hypothetical population of adults with a mean height of 160 cm.

Standard deviation (SD): If the standard deviation is 10 cm, approximately 68% of the population's heights fall between 150 and 170 cm (mean ± 1 SD), and about 95% fall between 140 and 180 cm (mean ± 2 SD).

Standard error (SE): If multiple random samples are taken from this population, their means will vary. The standard error estimates how much these sample means deviate from the true population mean of 160 cm. For instance, if the standard error is 2 cm, we can be approximately 95% confident that the true population mean lies between 156 and 164 cm (mean ± 1.96 SE).

Conceptual Questions

1. Define standard deviation (SD) and standard error (SE). How do these two measures differ in terms of what they represent in a dataset?
2. Describe the relationship between standard deviation and standard error. How is standard

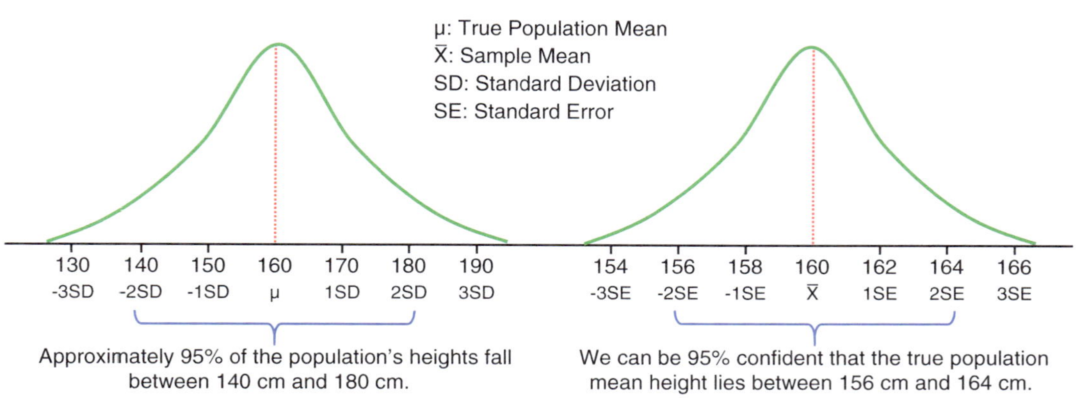

Fig. 11.2 Standard deviation vs. standard error

error calculated from standard deviation, and what does this relationship imply?
3. What percentage of the population falls within one and two standard deviations from the mean?
4. Explain how standard error is used to construct confidence intervals. Using the provided example, how would you calculate a 95% confidence interval for the true population mean based on the standard error?
5. How does sample size affect standard error? Discuss why larger sample sizes lead to smaller standard errors and the implications for research studies.

11.3 Type I Error, Type II Error, Power

The null hypothesis, denoted by H_0, is a statement asserting that there is no effect, no difference, or no relationship between certain variables in the population being studied. It serves as a default assumption, suggesting that any observed effect in the data is due to random chance. In contrast, the alternative hypothesis, denoted by H_1, contradicts the null hypothesis by proposing that there is an effect, a difference, or a relationship between the variables being studied.

H_0: Null hypothesis: Drug A and drug B have equal effects.

H_1: Alternative hypothesis: Drug A and drug B have different effects.

Type I Error (α)

A type I error occurs when we incorrectly *reject* a *true* null hypothesis. In other words, we conclude that there is a difference between drug A and drug B when, in fact, there is no difference, as illustrated in Table 11.1. Type I error is often referred to as a *false positive*.

Type II Error (β)

A type II error occurs when we *fail* to reject a *false* null hypothesis. In other words, we conclude that there is no difference between drug A and drug B when, in fact, there is a difference, as shown in Table 11.1.

Power (1 − β)

Power is the probability of *correctly* rejecting a *false* null hypothesis. It measures the *ability* of a statistical test to detect a *true* difference when one exists. Power ranges from 0 to 1. A power of 0 means the test will never correctly detect a true difference. A power of 1 means the test will always correctly detect a true difference. Power is complementary to type II error: power = $1 - \beta$.

Figure 11.3 illustrates the inverse relationship between type I error (α), type II error (β), and sample size in statistical hypothesis testing. On the left side, as type I error (indicated by the red arrow) increases, type II error (represented by the green arrow) decreases, demonstrating the trade-off between these two types of errors. Conversely, on the right side, an increase in sample size (shown by the blue arrow) leads to a decrease in

Table 11.1 Possible outcomes of a randomized trial: type I and type II errors

		Reality: Treatments are not different	Reality: Treatments are different
Our Conclusion	Treatments are not different	Correct Conclusion	Type II (α) Error
	Treatments are different	Type I (α) Error	Correct Conclusion

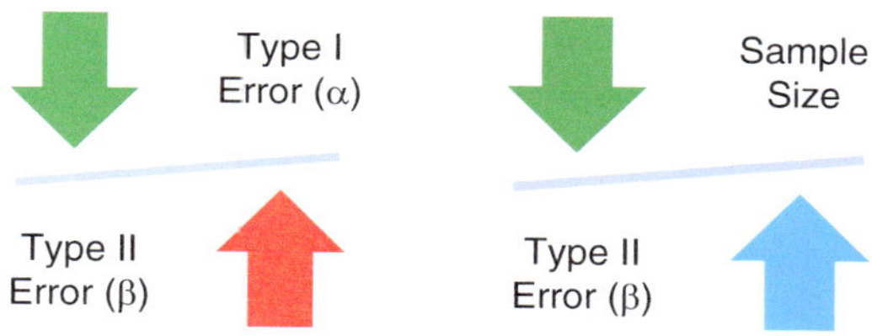

Fig. 11.3 Relationship between type I and type II errors and sample size

type II error (indicated by the green arrow). This highlights the importance of adequate sample size in reducing the likelihood of failing to reject a false null hypothesis (type II error).

Table 11.2 Factors affecting type I error (alpha), type II error (beta), and power

Factors	Type I error (α)	Type II error	Power ($1-\beta$)
Lowering significance level (alpha)	Decreases	Increases	Decreases
Increase sample size	No direct effect (at a fixed α level)	Decreases	Increases
Larger effect size	No direct effect (at a fixed α level)	Decreases	Increases
Less variability	No direct effect (at a fixed α level)	Decreases	Increases

Factors Affecting Type I Error, Type II Error, and Power

Type I and type II errors have an inverse relationship, meaning that reducing one often increases the other (when sample size, effect size, and variability are held constant). Additionally, power is directly related to type II error: As power increases, type II error decreases. Key factors influencing these errors are summarized in Table 11.2 [88].

The explanations for the factors presented in Table 11.2 that influence type I error (α), type II error (β), and power ($1-\beta$) are provided below.

Lowering Significance Level (Alpha)

- Type I error (α): Decreases because you reduce the chance of falsely rejecting a true null hypothesis, as you are requiring stronger evidence to make such a rejection.
- Type II error (β): Increases because a lower alpha level makes it harder to reject the null hypothesis, even when it is false, increasing the risk of failing to detect a true effect.
- Power ($1-\beta$): Decreases because power is the probability of correctly rejecting a false null hypothesis, and lowering alpha diminishes this probability. As type II error increases, power correspondingly decreases.

Increase Sample Size

- Type I error (α): No direct effect because α is predetermined by the researcher (although larger samples can indirectly make it more likely to get a p-value below the α level)
- Type II error (β): Decreases because larger sample sizes provide more information and increase the likelihood of detecting a true effect
- Power ($1-\beta$): Increases as a larger sample size improves the ability to detect an effect if it exists

Larger Effect Size

- Type I error (α): No direct effect because α depends on the threshold set by the researcher
- Type II error (β): Decreases because a larger effect size makes it easier to detect the effect
- Power ($1-\beta$): Increases since a larger effect size increases the likelihood of correctly rejecting a false null hypothesis

Less Variability

- Type I error (α): No direct effect since variability does not influence the chosen α level
- Type II error (β): Decreases because less variability in the data makes it easier to detect true effects
- Power ($1-\beta$): Increases as reduced variability improves the ability to detect an effect

In summary, type I error and *validity* are closely related concepts that impact the *accuracy* of research. A high rate of type I errors diminishes the validity of a study by increasing the likelihood of false positives. Conversely, validity is a broader concept that encompasses the overall accuracy of a study, including its ability to measure what it intends to measure, which involves avoiding both false positives and false negatives.

Relationship Between Sample Size and Type I Error Rate

Increasing the sample size does not directly affect the type I error rate (α) itself, as α is predetermined by the researcher. Conversely, when researchers choose a lower significance level (e.g., from 0.05 to 0.01), they effectively reduce the probability of making a type I error. To maintain the same power ($1 - \beta$) of the test—meaning the ability to detect a true effect if one exists—researchers may need to increase the sample size. A lower α requires more stringent evidence to reject the null hypothesis, which can necessitate a larger sample to achieve statistical significance. Power calculations before data collection are therefore essential to balance α, β, sample size, and effect size.

Conceptual Questions

1. What is the significance of the null hypothesis in the context of statistical testing, and why is it often referred to as the "default" assumption?
2. Define type I error and type II error in the context of hypothesis testing. How do these errors relate to the null hypothesis (H_0) and alternative hypothesis (H_1)?
3. What are the potential consequences of committing a type I error in a clinical trial? Discuss how this might affect patient safety, treatment protocols, and future research.
4. Explain the implications of a type II error in a clinical trial. How might this error affect the perception of a drug's effectiveness and the decisions made based on the trial results?
5. How does lowering the significance level (alpha) impact type I error and power? Why might researchers choose to set a lower alpha level in certain studies?
6. Explain how increasing the sample size influences type II error and power. Why is a larger sample size beneficial in hypothesis testing?

12 The Concept of Causality in Epidemiology

Contents

12.1 The Foundations of Causality

Causality is a core concept in epidemiology, enabling researchers to identify the causes of diseases and their effects on populations. It describes the relationship between an event (the cause) and a subsequent outcome (the effect), where the former directly influences the latter. A clear understanding of causality is essential for designing effective public health interventions and policies to prevent diseases and improve health outcomes.

Causality in Epidemiological Research

Epidemiologists use various study designs to explore causality, each with its strengths and limitations.

Experimental Studies

Randomized controlled trials (RCTs) are considered the *gold standard* for establishing causality. In an RCT, participants are randomly assigned to an intervention group or a control group. This randomization minimizes bias and confounding, allowing researchers to attribute observed effects to the intervention.

Observational Studies

When experiments are not feasible or ethical, observational studies provide valuable insights. These include:

- Cohort studies: Follow groups of individuals over time to compare the incidence of outcomes between those exposed and unexposed to a factor.
- Case-control studies: Compare individuals with a disease (cases) to those without it (controls) to identify potential exposures.
- Cross-sectional studies: Examine exposure and outcome at a single point in time.

While observational studies are prone to confounding and bias, techniques such as stratification and multivariable analysis help address these challenges.

J. Poorolajal, *Illustrated Epidemiology*, https://doi.org/10.1007/978-981-96-9566-9_12

Challenges in Establishing Causality

Epidemiologists encounter numerous challenges when studying causality, necessitating careful study design, rigorous analysis, and transparent reporting. Key challenges include:

- Confounding: This occurs when a third variable influences both the exposure and the outcome, leading to a misleading association.
- Information bias: Systematic errors in measuring either the exposure or the outcome can lead to incorrect conclusions about the relationship between them.
- Selection bias: Findings from a study may not be applicable to broader populations if the sample is not representative, limiting the ability to infer causality.
- Random error: In studies involving rare exposures or outcomes, small sample sizes increase the likelihood of random error, leading to imprecise estimates and reduced statistical power. This can obscure true associations or suggest spurious ones, complicating causal inference.
- Temporal ambiguity: Establishing a clear timeline of exposure and outcome is crucial; however, in some studies, the timing may be unclear, complicating causal interpretations.
- Reverse causation: In some cases, the outcome may influence the exposure rather than the reverse, complicating the determination of causality.

To address these complexities, epidemiology relies on various theories to conceptualize causality, each providing a structured approach to understanding disease etiology. The main theories are outlined in the following sections.

12.2 Austin Bradford Hill's Criteria

In the twentieth century, Austin Bradford Hill outlined key criteria—often called Hill's criteria—to help establish causation in epidemiological studies [89]. These criteria provide a structured way to assess potential causal links, though not all criteria need to be met for causation to be inferred. These include (Fig. 12.1):

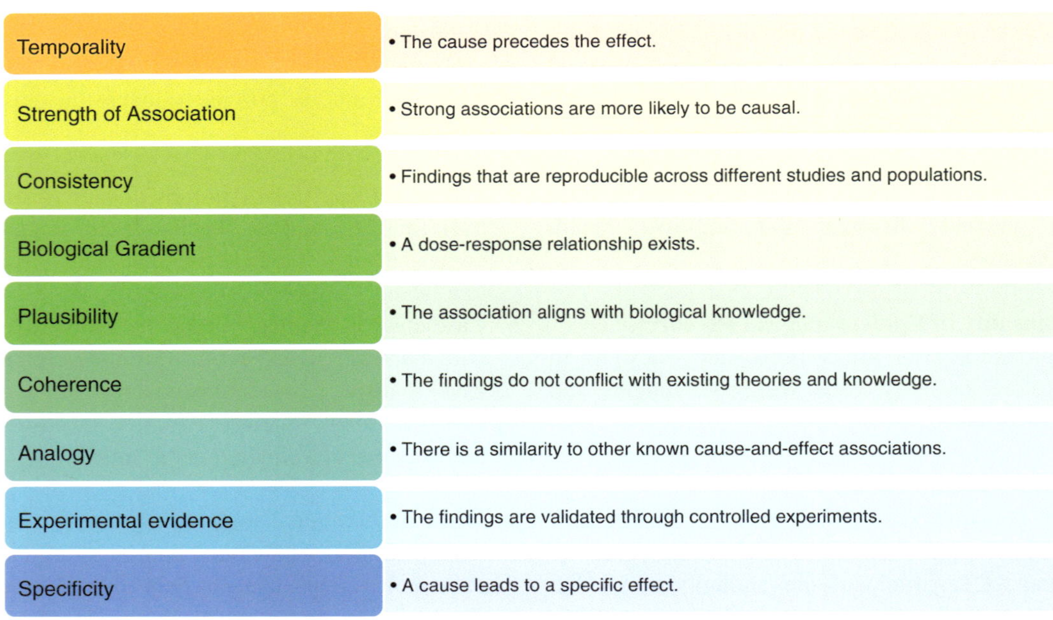

Fig. 12.1 Bradford Hill's criteria for causation in epidemiology

Temporality

As illustrated in Fig. 12.2, temporality refers to the essential principle that a cause must always precede its effect in time. In other words, exposure always precedes the outcome. This criterion is fundamental and indisputable; it is imperative for a cause to occur before its effect. The absence of this temporal sequence serves as strong evidence against the notion of causality.

A lack of sufficient information regarding the temporal sequence between exposure and outcome can lead to *reverse causality*. Reverse causality occurs when the direction of cause and effect in a relationship is opposite to what is assumed; instead of the exposure causing the outcome, the outcome influences the exposure. This can result in incorrect conclusions about the nature of the association if not properly accounted for in the study design or analysis. To address reverse causality, researchers often employ longitudinal studies, temporal data, or sensitivity analyses to clarify the sequence of events.

Example 1

A study may find that individuals who are physically inactive are more likely to have chronic illnesses, such as heart disease. While it might appear that inactivity causes heart disease, reverse causality could occur if the chronic illness itself limits the individual's ability to engage in physical activity.

Example 2

A study might find that individuals with depression are more likely to be unemployed. While it may seem that unemployment causes depression, the relationship could also work in reverse—depression might reduce a person's ability to perform at work, leading to unemployment.

Strength of Association

As illustrated in Fig. 12.3, strong associations are generally more indicative of causality than weak associations, with strength measured by metrics such as the risk ratio (RR), where an RR greater than 2.0 is often deemed strong [4]. For example, the combined effect of hepatitis B virus (HBV) and hepatitis C virus (HCV) increases the likelihood of developing hepatocellular carcinoma (HCC) by 32.58 times compared to individuals who do not have these infections [90]. Such a strong association suggests a causal relationship. However, a weak association does not exclude the possibility of a causal connection. Importantly, a strong association is neither a necessary nor sufficient condition for causality, just as a weak association does not definitively indicate a lack of causality.

Consistency

Consistency, as illustrated in Fig. 12.4, refers to the repeated observation of a specific association or effect across different studies, populations, settings, and methodologies. In epidemiological research, a consistent finding strengthens the evidence for a causal relationship, as it suggests that the association is not due to chance, bias, or confounding factors. However, a lack of consistency does not necessarily negate a causal relationship, as some effects may only arise under specific or unusual conditions. For example, while tampon use can lead to toxic shock syndrome, this occurs only rarely, illustrating that even infrequent associations can still be causal [91].

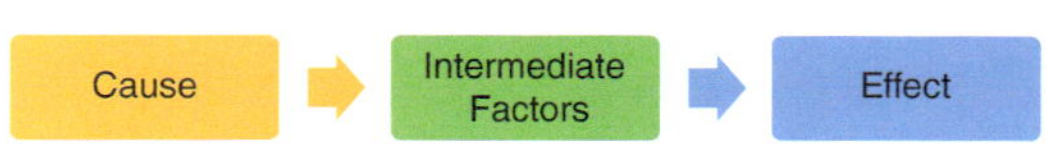

Fig. 12.2 Temporality—the cause always precedes the effect

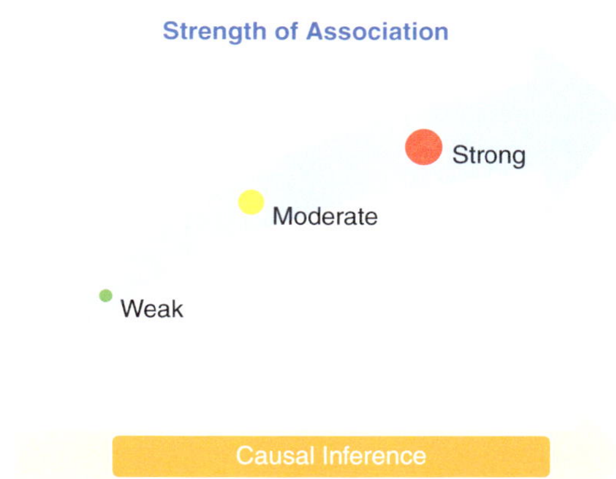

Fig. 12.3 Strength of association and its role in causal inference

Biological Gradient

A biological gradient, also known as a *dose-response* relationship, refers to the observation that as the level of exposure to a risk factor increases, the risk of a specific outcome or disease also increases. This relationship suggests that higher doses of exposure are associated with a greater likelihood of the outcome or disease. For instance, as illustrated in Fig. 12.5, as a woman smokes more cigarettes during pregnancy, her risk of having a low-birth-weight baby increases. This illustrates a clear biological gradient, where the intensity of exposure (cigarette smoking) correlates with the severity of the outcome (low birth weight) [2].

Plausibility

Plausibility refers to the degree to which an observed association between a potential cause and an effect can be reasonably explained by existing biological knowledge and mechanisms. An association is considered biologically believable when it aligns with established scientific understanding. For example, as illustrated in Fig. 12.6, the link between cigarette smoking and lung cancer is plausible because it is supported by well-documented biological mechanisms that explain how smoking can lead to cancer development.

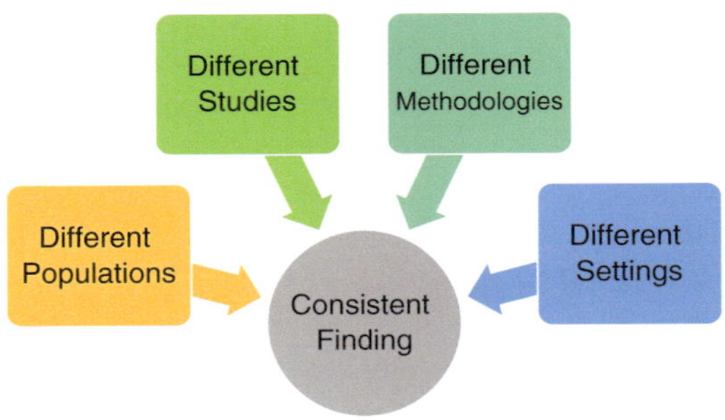

Fig. 12.4 Demonstrating consistency of findings across diverse contexts

Coherence

Coherence means that the observed association does not conflict with existing knowledge of the disease's natural history and biology. In other words, the evidence fits with the broader understanding of the topic. It implies that evidence for a causal relationship should align with established facts about the disease and its causes, meaning the association should not contradict known biological and clinical evidence. Coherence strengthens causal arguments by ensuring that proposed links are compatible with known biological processes. The absence of coherence does not necessarily negate causality, nor does its presence guarantee it.

The distinction between plausibility and coherence is subtle yet significant. Plausibility is framed *positively*, suggesting that an association *should* align with established scientific knowledge and have a logical biological explanation. In contrast, coherence is expressed *negatively*, emphasizing that an association *should not*

Fig. 12.5 Percentage of pregnancies with infants weighing less than 2500 g by maternal cigarette smoking category

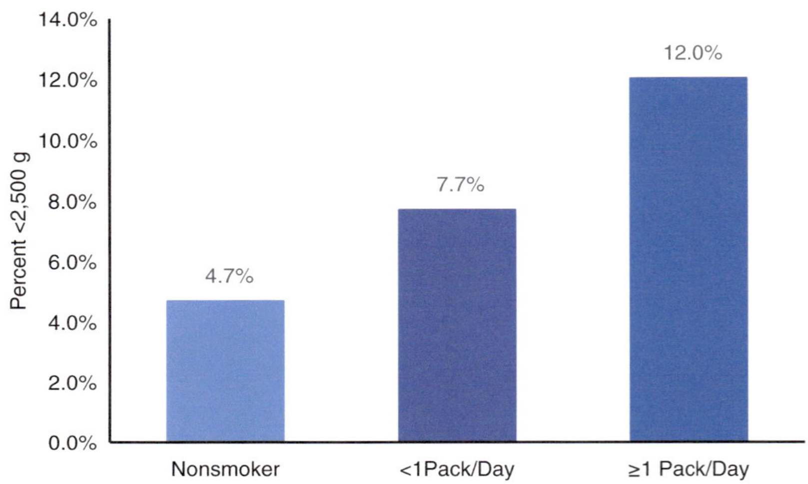

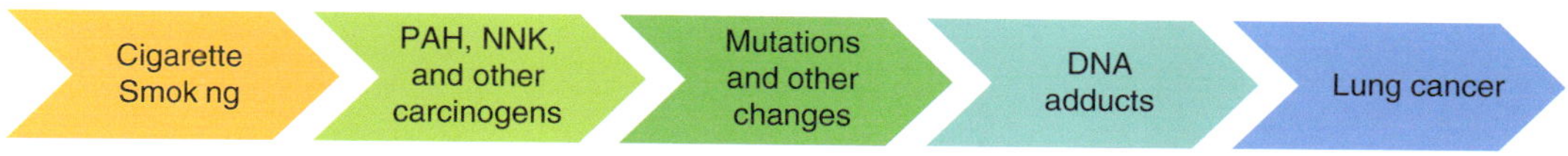

Fig. 12.6 Biological mechanisms linking smoking to cancer development (PAH, polycyclic aromatic hydrocarbons; NNK, nicotine-derived nitrosamine ketone)

contradict existing knowledge about the disease and its mechanisms.

Analogy

An analogy refers to drawing comparisons between two situations or phenomena to infer causal relationships based on similarities in their properties or patterns. This method relies on the assumption that if two situations share similar characteristics and one is known to cause an effect, the same causal relationship may exist in the other situation.

Example 3

As illustrated in Fig. 12.7, consider the well-established causal link between smoking and lung cancer, which is supported by extensive research. Now, suppose we want to investigate the potential causal relationship between marijuana and lung cancer. We can draw an analogy between these two situations to explore whether similar effects might occur.

Example 4

The established risk of skin cancer from UV radiation due to sun exposure prompts researchers to investigate whether tanning beds, which emit similar types of UV radiation, pose a comparable risk for developing skin cancer. This analogy guides further research into the safety and health implications of artificial tanning methods.

Example 5

The known causal link between chronic hepatitis B infection and liver cancer is analogous to the role of HPV in causing cervical cancer, as both involve persistent viral infections leading to malignancy.

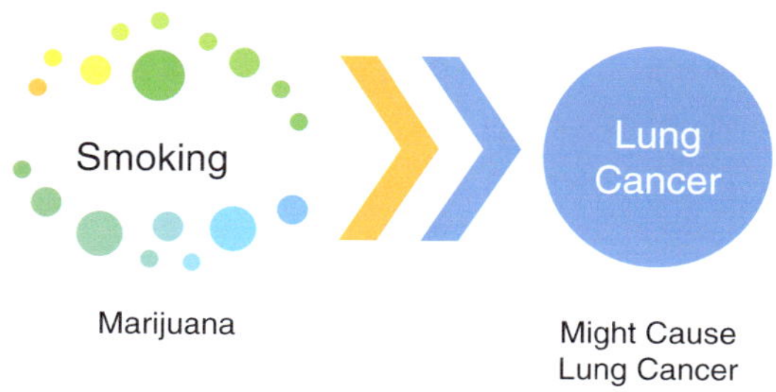

Fig. 12.7 Analogy of the associations between smoking and lung cancer compared to marijuana and lung cancer

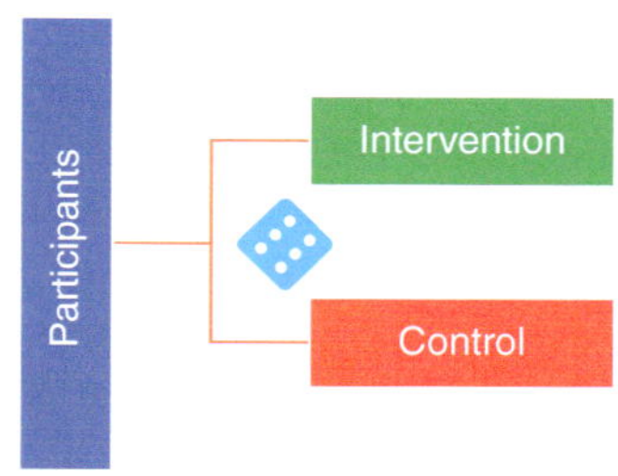

Fig. 12.8 Randomized controlled trial (RCT) as evidence for causal inference

Experimental Evidence

Experimental evidence for causal inference refers to data obtained from controlled experiments designed to determine causal relationships by manipulating an independent variable and observing its effect on a dependent variable. In epidemiology, as illustrated in Fig. 12.8, a classic example is a randomized controlled trial (RCT) where researchers might randomly assign participants to receive a new vaccine (the independent variable) or a placebo (the control) to observe the vaccine's effect on the incidence of a specific disease (the dependent variable). If the group receiving the vaccine experiences significantly fewer

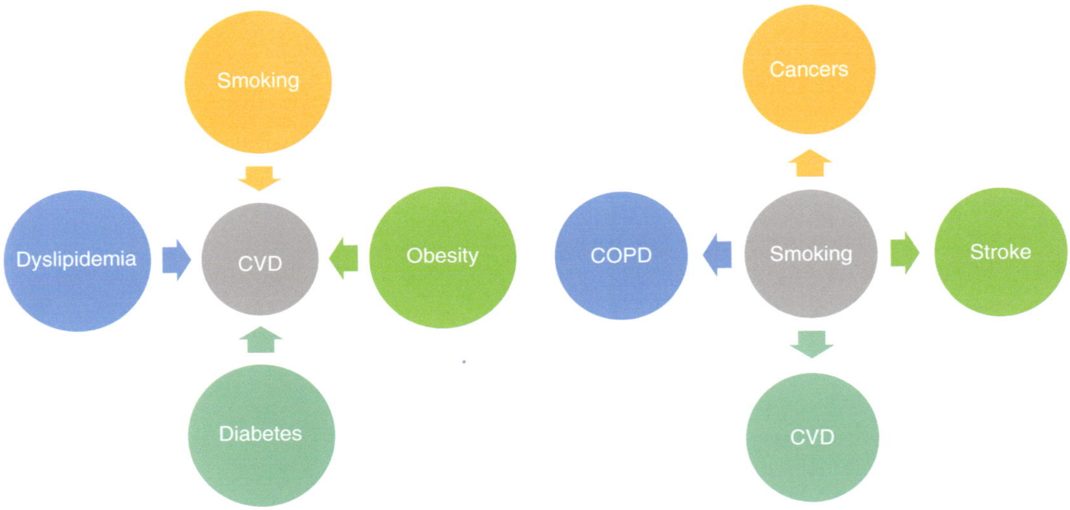

Fig. 12.9 Counterexamples to specificity: one exposure with multiple outcomes and multiple risk factors for a single outcome (CVD, cardiovascular disease; COPD, chronic obstructive pulmonary disease)

cases of disease, it provides strong experimental evidence supporting the causal inference that the vaccine is effective in preventing that disease.

Specificity

Specificity in causal inference refers to the idea that a particular exposure is associated with a single, specific outcome or that a specific outcome is caused by a single exposure. It strengthens causal arguments by demonstrating a clear and unique relationship between the exposure and the effect. However, in complex diseases with multiple risk factors and outcomes, specificity is often difficult to establish and is considered less applicable in modern epidemiology.

The relationship between *Mycobacterium tuberculosis* infection and tuberculosis (TB) is an example of specificity. This relationship is highly specific because the *Mycobacterium tuberculosis* bacterium is the primary cause of TB, and TB rarely occurs in the absence of this specific pathogen.

While specificity can support causality, it is not always necessary. As illustrated in Fig. 12.9, many chronic diseases (e.g., cardiovascular disease) have multiple risk factors, and a single exposure (e.g., smoking) can contribute to multiple outcomes (e.g., lung cancer, heart disease, and stroke).

12.3 The Sufficient-Component Cause Model

The sufficient-component cause model, often visualized as the "causal pie model," is a framework in epidemiology that describes how multiple factors work together to produce a specific outcome. Proposed by Kenneth J. Rothman, it emphasizes the multifactorial nature of causation and is widely used to understand the interplay between various factors in the development of diseases [7].

Key Components of the Theory

Sufficient Cause: A sufficient cause is a complete set of factors that, when present together, inevitably lead to the occurrence of a specific outcome. Each sufficient cause can be thought of as a "causal pie" made up of several contributing factors.

Necessary Cause: A necessary cause is a specific component that is part of every sufficient cause for a particular outcome. Without it, the outcome cannot occur.

Component Cause: Each factor in the pie is a component cause. These are the individual exposures or conditions that contribute to the outcome. A component cause alone is not enough to

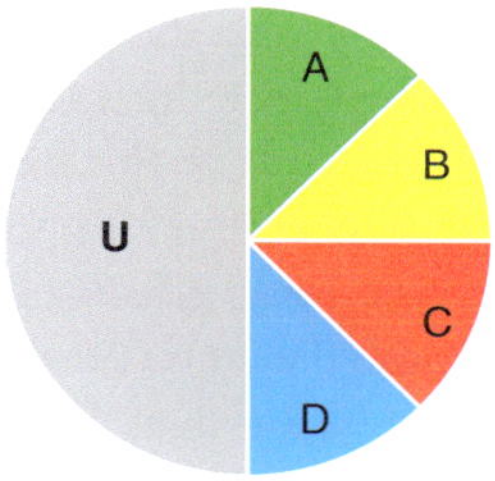

Fig. 12.10 Sufficient-component causes contributing to the development of tuberculosis

cause the outcome but works in combination with other factors.

Imagine the development of tuberculosis as the outcome. As illustrated in Fig. 12.10, a constellation of component causes forms a sufficient cause for tuberculosis:

- Component A: Presence of *Mycobacterium tuberculosis* (necessary cause)
- Component B: Malnutrition (component cause)
- Component C: Weakened immune system, such as that caused by HIV infection (component cause)
- Component D: Poor living conditions, including overcrowding and inadequate ventilation (component cause)
- Component U: Unmeasured or unknown factors that may also contribute to the risk of developing TB (unknown component cause)

Implications for Public Health

The sufficient-component cause model underscores the necessity of addressing multiple factors to effectively prevent disease. This model emphasizes that diseases often result from a combination of various components rather than a single cause, highlighting the complexity of disease etiology. In the context of tuberculosis (TB), this understanding can inform a range of targeted interventions designed to mitigate risk and enhance health outcomes. Key interventions could include:

- Improving housing and ventilation: Overcrowding and poor housing conditions are significant risk factors for TB transmission. Public health efforts should focus on enhancing housing quality and ensuring adequate ventilation in living spaces to reduce the risk of airborne transmission.
- Strengthening healthcare access: Ensuring that at-risk populations, such as individuals living with HIV, have access to healthcare services is essential for the early detection and treatment of TB.
- Enhancing nutrition and immune function: Addressing nutritional deficiencies in at-risk populations can significantly improve immune function, making individuals less susceptible to infections like TB. Public health initiatives could include nutritional education and food assistance programs to improve access to healthy foods.

The sufficient-component cause model provides a structured framework for understanding how complex interactions among various factors lead to health outcomes. By recognizing the multifaceted nature of disease causation, public health professionals can design and implement comprehensive interventions that disrupt the pathways to disease, ultimately improving public health outcomes and reducing the burden of tuberculosis.

12.4 The Equivalence Model

The equivalence model for causal inference is a novel graphical framework designed to integrate both *risk* factors and *protective* factors in determining the likelihood of an outcome, such as disease development. Proposed by Jalal Poorolajal, this model provides a more comprehensive perspective by balancing these opposing influences, offering insights into cases where traditional models may fail to explain causation [92].

The model addresses a key challenge in epidemiology of understanding why some high-risk individuals, such as heavy smokers with a long history of smoking, may not develop diseases like lung cancer, while some low-risk individuals, such as low or nonsmokers, may. To tackle this issue, the equivalence model visually represents the combined effects of risk and protective factors at the individual level. Risk factors promote disease development, while protective factors inhibit it. The model illustrates that when there is a balance between these factors, the disease will not occur; specifically, if the overall weight of risk factors is less than or equal to that of protective factors, the outcome will not happen. Conversely, if the weight of risk factors exceeds that of protective factors, the disease will occur.

Figure 12.11 illustrates the simplest form of the equivalence model for a hypothetical disease (e.g., hypertension) influenced by a single risk factor (e.g., salt intake) and a single protective factor (e.g., physical activity). In this scenario, a balance exists between the levels of exposure to the risk and protective factors. Neither factor can overpower the other; therefore, the outcome (hypertension) will not occur.

However, in real life, multiple risk factors (e.g., salt intake, stress, smoking, alcohol consumption, family history) and protective factors (e.g., physical activity, maintaining a healthy weight, following a nutritious diet, adequate potassium intake) influence the development of any specific disease, such as hypertension. These risk and protective factors interact with one another in complex ways. As illustrated in Fig. 12.12, a disease will not develop until there is an imbalance between the levels of exposure to risk and protective factors. Regardless of the number and level of risk and protective factors involved, as well as their interactions, the outcome ultimately depends on this balance.

As illustrated in Fig. 12.13, an imbalance exists between the overall effects of risk and protective factors, with the cumulative weight of the risk factors being greater than that of the protective factors. Consequently, this imbalance leads to the occurrence of the outcome (e.g., disease).

As illustrated in Fig. 12.14, an imbalance exists between the overall effects of risk and protective factors, with the cumulative weight of the protective factors exceeding that of the risk factors. Consequently, this imbalance prevents the development of the disease, even though several risk factors play a role in this model.

Significance

The model addresses limitations in causality analysis by explicitly incorporating protective factors alongside risk factors, providing a more comprehensive understanding of disease dynamics. The equivalence model helps explain why, for instance, a moderate smoker or even a nonsmoker may develop lung cancer, while a heavy smoker may remain unaffected. The critical relationship lies in the balance between the overall effects of known and unknown risk factors that predispose an individual to the disease and the known and unknown protective factors that help prevent it. If the cumulative weight of risk factors exceeds that of protective factors, the disease

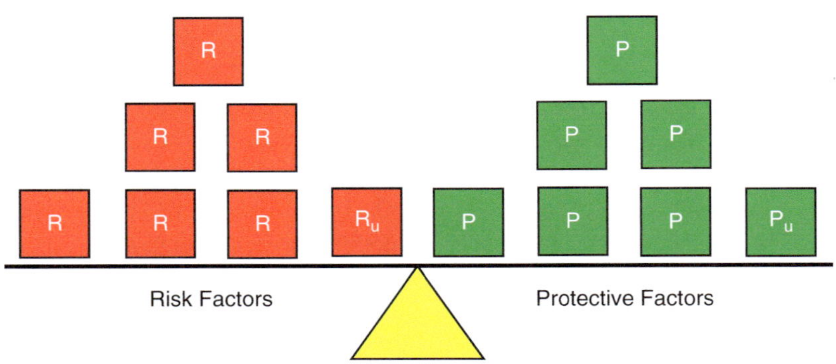

Fig. 12.11 Equivalence model for a hypothetical single risk and protective factors. In this model, the risk factor is denoted by R and the protective factor by P, while unknown risk and protective factors are represented by R_U and P_U, respectively. The number of shapes (squares) indicates the level of exposure; more shapes represent higher levels of exposure. A balance exists between the effects of risk and protective factors

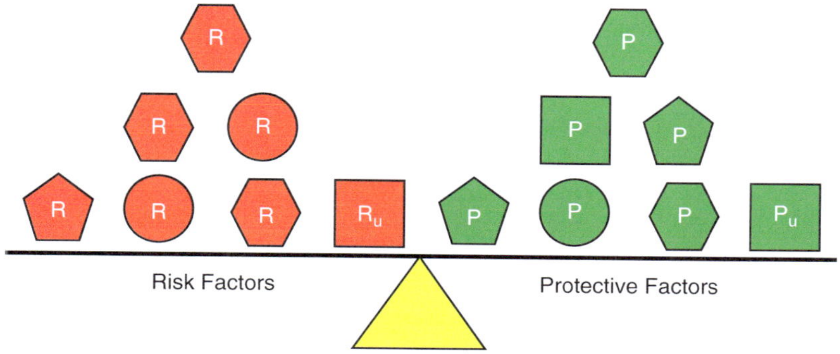

Fig. 12.12 Equivalence model for multiple risk and protective factors. In this model, risk factors are denoted by R and protective factors by P, while unknown risk and protective factors are represented by R_U and P_U, respectively. Different shapes (circles, squares, pentagons, or hexagons) indicate various risk or protective factors, with the repetition of each shape representing the level of exposure. A balance exists between the overall effects of risk factors, protective factors, and their interactions

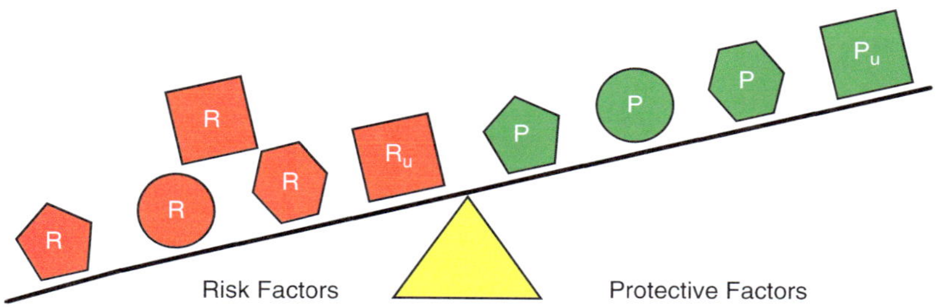

Fig. 12.13 Equivalence model for multiple risk and protective factors. In this model, risk factors are denoted by R, while protective factors are represented by P. Unknown risk and protective factors are indicated by R_U and P_U, respectively. Different shapes—such as circles, squares, pentagons, or hexatones—represent various risk or protective factors, with the repetition of each shape reflecting the level of exposure. An imbalance exists between the overall effects of risk factors and protective factors, with the overall effect of the risk factors surpassing that of the protective factors

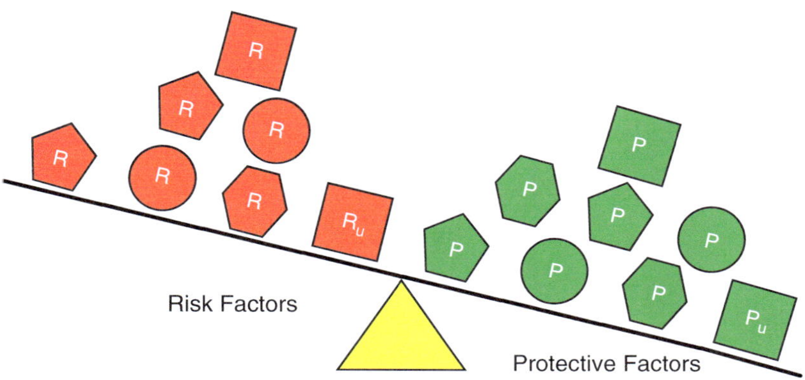

Fig. 12.14 Equivalence model for multiple risk and protective factors. In this model, risk factors are denoted by R, while protective factors are represented by P. Unknown risk and protective factors are indicated by R_U and P_U, respectively. Different shapes—such as circles, squares, pentagons, or hexatones—represent various risk or protective factors, with the repetition of each shape reflecting the level of exposure. An imbalance exists between the overall effects of risk factors and protective factors, with the overall effect of the protective factors overwhelming that of the risk factors

(e.g., lung cancer) will develop. Conversely, if the cumulative weight of protective factors is greater than that of risk factors, the disease will not develop. This balance-oriented framework is particularly relevant in epidemiology and health policy, where interventions often focus on modifying protective factors to mitigate risks.

Conceptual Questions

1. How does the concept of causality in epidemiology differ from everyday understandings of cause and effect? Why is it important to have a precise definition in the context of public health?
2. Discuss the significance of each of Bradford Hill's criteria for causation. Which criteria do you think is the most critical in establishing a causal relationship, and why?
3. Describe the sufficient-component cause model. How does this model enhance our understanding of multifactorial diseases compared to a single-cause model?
4. Discuss how the equivalence model integrates risk and protective factors. Why is this integration important for understanding disease outcomes?
5. Based on the equivalence model, what strategies might public health officials consider to prevent diseases in high-risk populations? How can they leverage protective factors effectively?
6. How can the concepts of causality discussed in this chapter be applied to present public health challenges, such as the COVID-19 pandemic or obesity?

References

1. Porta M. A dictionary of epidemiology. New York: Oxford University Press; 2014.
2. Celentano DD, Szklo M. Gordis epidemiology. 6th ed. Philadelphia: Elsevier Inc; 2019.
3. Sackett DL, Haynes RB, Tugnell P. Clinical epidemiology, a basic science for clinical medicine. 4th ed. Boston: Little, Brown and Company; 2014.
4. Bonita R, Beaglehole R, Kjellström T. Basic epidemiology. 2nd ed. Geneva: WHO; 2006.
5. Pahkala K, Hietalampi H, Laitinen TT, Viikari JS, Rönnemaa T, Niinikoski H, et al. Ideal cardiovascular health in adolescence: effect of lifestyle intervention and association with vascular intima-media thickness and elasticity (the Special Turku Coronary Risk Factor Intervention Project for Children [STRIP] study). Circulation. 2013;127:2088–96.
6. Falkner B, Lurbe E. Primordial prevention of high blood pressure in childhood: an opportunity not to be missed. Hypertension. 2020;75:1142–50.
7. Lash TL, VanderWeele TJ, Haneuse S, Rothman KJ. Modern epidemiology. 4th ed. Philadelphia: Wolters Kluwer; 2021.
8. Szklo M, Nieto FJ. Epidemiology: beyond the basics. 4th ed. Burlington: Jones & Bartlett Learning; 2019.
9. United Nations. World population day. New York: UN; 2024. [cited 6 December 2024]; Available from: https://www.un.org/en/observances/world-population-day
10. World Health Organization. Key facts HIV. Geneva: WHO; 2022.
11. Center for Disease Control and Prevention. Stroke facts. Atlanta: CDC; 2024. [updated 24 October, 2024; cited 6 December 2024]; Available from: https://www.cdc.gov/stroke/data-research/facts-stats/index.html
12. Menachemi N, Yiannoutsos CT, Dixon BE, Duszynski TJ, Fadel WF, Wools-Kaloustian KK, et al. Population point prevalence of SARS-CoV-2 infection based on a statewide random sample – Indiana, April 25–29, 2020. MMWR Morb Mortal Wkly Rep. 2020;69:960–4.
13. Guerra FM, Bolotin S, Lim G, Heffernan J, Deeks SL, Li Y, et al. The basic reproduction number (R(0)) of measles: a systematic review. Lancet Infect Dis. 2017;17:e420–e8.
14. Mazaheri S, Poorolajal J, Mazaheri A. Sensitivity and specificity of Electrodiagnostic parameters in diagnosing carpal tunnel syndrome: a case-control study. Bone Joint Open. 2024;5:898–903.
15. Farimani M, Poorolajal J, Rabiee S, Bahmanzadeh M. Successful pregnancy and live birth after intrauterine Administration of Autologous Platelet-Rich Plasma in a woman with recurrent implantation failure: a case report. Int J Reprod Biomed. 2017;15:803–6.
16. Kannan L, Bauman AA. Purple urine in a patient with UTI and constipation. Oxf Med Case Rep. 2023;2023:omad013.
17. Pieretti VM, Agriello M, Molina MMD, Bonaura P, Ramallo CA, Miraglia E, et al. Monkeypox: case series. Rev Fac Cien Med Univ Nac Cordoba. 2023;80:321–34.
18. Markman TM, Hamilton RH, Marchlinski FE, Nazarian S. Case series of transcutaneous magnetic stimulation for ventricular tachycardia storm. JAMA. 2020;323:2200–2.
19. Poorolajal J, Ahmadpoor J, Mohammadi Y, Soltanian AR, Asghari SZ, Mazloumi E. Prevalence of problematic internet use disorder and associated risk factors and complications among Iranian University students: a national survey. Health Promot Perspect. 2019;9:207–13.
20. Shahbazi F, Zareie B, Poorolajal J. The association between socio-economic inequality and the global prevalence of anxiety and depressive disorders: an ecological study. Gen Psychiatr. 2022;35:e100735.
21. Messerli FH. Chocolate consumption, cognitive function, and Nobel laureates. N Engl J Med. 2012;367:1562–4.
22. Morgenstern H. Ecologic studies in epidemiology: concepts, principles, and methods. Annu Rev Public Health. 1995;16:61–81.
23. Taheri-Kharameh Z, Poorolajal J, Bashirian S, Heydari Moghadam R, Parham M, Barati M, et al. Risk factors for falls in Iranian older adults: a case-control study. Int J Inj Control Saf Promot. 2019;26:354–9.

J. Poorolajal. *Illustrated Epidemiology*, https://doi.org/10.1007/978-981-96-9566-9

24. Langholz B, Thomas DC. Nested case-control and case-cohort methods of sampling from a cohort: a critical comparison. Am J Epidemiol. 1990;131:169–76.
25. Ernster VL. Nested case-control studies. Prev Med. 1994;23:587–90.
26. Hennekens CH, Buring JE. Methodologic considerations in the design and conduct of randomized trials: the U.S. Physicians' Health Study. Control Clin Trials. 1989;10:142s–50s.
27. Ridker PM, Cushman M, Stampfer MJ, Tracy RP, Hennekens CH. Inflammation, aspirin, and the risk of cardiovascular disease in apparently healthy men. N Engl J Med. 1997;336:973–9.
28. Grayson JK. Radiation exposure, socioeconomic status, and brain tumor risk in the US Air Force: a nested case-control study. Am J Epidemiol. 1996;143:480–6.
29. Poorolajal J, Alafchi B, Vosoogi RN, Hamzeh S, Ghahramani M. Risk factors for maternal mortality in the west of Iran: a nested case-control study. Epidemiol Health. 2014;36:e2014028.
30. Chu CS, Lee FL, Bai YM, Su TP, Tsai SJ, Chen TJ, et al. Antidepressant drugs use and epilepsy risk: a nationwide nested case-control study. Epilepsy Behav. 2023;140:109102.
31. Nieto FJ, Folsom AR, Sorlie PD, Grayston JT, Wang SP, Chambless LE. Chlamydia pneumoniae infection and incident coronary heart disease: the atherosclerosis risk in communities study. Am J Epidemiol. 1999;150:149–56.
32. Dekker JM, Crow RS, Folsom AR, Hannan PJ, Liao D, Swenne CA, et al. Low heart rate variability in a 2-minute rhythm Strip predicts risk of coronary heart disease and mortality from several causes: the ARIC Study. Atherosclerosis Risk in Communities. Circulation. 2000;102:1239–44.
33. Maclure M, Mittleman MA. Should we use a case-crossover design? Annu Rev Public Health. 2000;21:193–221.
34. Valent F, Brusaferro S, Barbone F. A case-crossover study of sleep and childhood injury. Pediatrics. 2001;107:E23.
35. Sornpaisarn B, Sornpaisarn S, Shield KD, Rehm J. Alcohol use and injury risk in Thailand: a case-crossover emergency department study. Drug Alcohol Rev. 2020;39:539–45.
36. Basu R, Pearson D, Sie L, Broadwin R. A case-crossover study of temperature and infant mortality in California. Paediatr Perinat Epidemiol. 2015;29:407–15.
37. Jovanovic N, Peek-Asa C, Zhang L, Cavanaugh JE, Pidro A, Alajbegovic-Halimic J. The risk and protective factors for pediatric eye injuries: a case-crossover study. Ophthalmic Epidemiol. 2021;28:479–87.
38. Dawber TR, Moore FE, Mann GV. Coronary heart disease in the Framingham Study. Am J Public Health Nations Health. 1957;47:4–24.
39. Kaslow RA, Ostrow DG, Detels R, Phair JP, Polk BF, Rinaldo CR Jr. The multicenter AIDS Cohort Study: rationale, organization, and selected characteristics of the participants. Am J Epidemiol. 1987;126:310–8.
40. Stampfer MJ, Willett WC, Colditz GA, Rosner B, Speizer FE, Hennekens CH. A prospective study of postmenopausal estrogen therapy and coronary heart disease. N Engl J Med. 1985;313:1044–9.
41. Ascherio A, Rimm EB, Stampfer MJ, Giovannucci EL, Willett WC. Dietary intake of marine N-3 fatty acids, fish intake, and the risk of coronary disease among men. N Engl J Med. 1995;332:977–82.
42. Pakrad F, Shiri R, Mozayani Monfared A, Mohammadi Saleh R, Poorolajal J. Predictors of premature mortality following coronary artery bypass grafting: an Iranian Single-Centre Study. Healthcare (Basel). 2023;12:36.
43. Li W, Chen D, Peng Y, Lu Z, Kwan MP, Tse LA. Association between metabolic syndrome and mortality: prospective cohort study. JMIR Public Health Surveill. 2023;9:e44073.
44. Zingel R, Jacob L, Smith L, Konrad M, Kostev K. Association between psoriasis and dementia: a retrospective cohort study. J Alzheimers Dis Rep. 2023;7:41–9.
45. Hashemian F, Ghorbanian MA, Jahanshahi J, Hashemian F, Poorolajal J. Effect of topical furosemide on Rhinosinusal polyposis relapse after endoscopic sinus surgery: a randomized clinical trial. JAMA Otolaryngol Head Neck Surg. 2016;142:1045–9.
46. Sheikh V, Mozaiani-Monfared A, Gharakhani M, Poorolajal J. Effect of vitamin D supplementation versus placebo on essential hypertension in patients with vitamin D deficiency: a double-blind randomized clinical trial. J Clin Hypertens. 2020;22:1867–73.
47. Masoumi SZ, Asl HR, Poorolajal J, Panah MH, Oliaei SR. Evaluation of mint efficacy regarding dysmenorrhea in comparison with Mefenamic acid: a double blinded randomized crossover study. Iran J Nurs Midwifery Res. 2016;21:363–7.
48. Hennekens CH, Buring JE, Manson JE, Stampfer M, Rosner B, Cook NR, et al. Lack of effect of long-term supplementation with Beta carotene on the incidence of malignant neoplasms and cardiovascular disease. N Engl J Med. 1996;334:1145–9.
49. Chow S-C, Liu J-P. Design and analysis of clinical trials: concepts and methodologies. 4th ed. New Jersey: John Wiley & Sons; 2021.
50. Borenstein M, Hedges LV, Higgins JPT, Rothstein HR. Introduction to meta-analysis. 2nd ed. Chichester: John Wiley & Sons, Ltd; 2021.
51. Higgins JPT, Thomas J, Chandler J, Cumpston M, Li T, Page MJ, et al. Cochrane handbook for systematic reviews of interventions. Cochrane; 2023. Available from: www.training.cochrane.org/handbook
52. Compérat E, Amin MB, Cathomas R, Choudhury A, De Santis M, Kamat A, et al. Current best practice for bladder cancer: a narrative review of diagnostics and treatments. Lancet. 2022;400:1712–21.
53. Khangura S, Konnyu K, Cushman R, Grimshaw J, Moher D. Evidence summaries: the evolution of a rapid review approach. Syst Rev. 2012;1:10.
54. Brooks SK, Webster RK, Smith LE, Woodland L, Wessely S, Greenberg N, et al. The psychological

impact of quarantine and how to reduce it: rapid review of the evidence. Lancet. 2020;395:912–20.
55. Peters MD, Godfrey CM, Khalil H, McInerney P, Parker D, Soares CB. Guidance for conducting systematic scoping reviews. Int J Evid Based Healthc. 2015;13:141–6.
56. Alrubaian F, Mulla Z. Governments policy measures to address obesity among adults: a scoping review of the global evidence. Lancet. 2023;402(Suppl 1):S20.
57. Center for Reviews and Dissemination. Systematic reviews: CRD'S guidance for undertaking reviews in health care. New York: CRD; 2009.
58. Rashti R, Ghasemi F, Poorolajal J. Association between birth weight and risk of nonneurological childhood cancers: a systematic review and meta-analysis. Eur J Cancer Prev. 2025;34:40–52.
59. Choi GJ, Kang H. Introduction to umbrella reviews as a useful evidence-based practice. J Lipid Atheroscler. 2023;12:3–11.
60. Singh M, Wambua S, Lee SI, Okoth K, Wang Z, Fazla F, et al. Autoimmune diseases and adverse pregnancy outcomes: an umbrella review. Lancet. 2023;402(Suppl 1):S84.
61. Petitti DB. Meta-analysis, decision analysis, and cost-effectiveness analysis: methods for quantitative synthesis in medicine. 2nd ed. Oxford: Oxford University Press; 2000.
62. Darvishi N, Poorolajal J, Azmi-Naei B, Farhadi M. The role of social support in preventing suicidal ideations and behaviors: a systematic review and meta-analysis. J Res Health Sci. 2024;24:e00609.
63. Salanti G, Del Giovane C, Chaimani A, Caldwell DM, Higgins JP. Evaluating the quality of evidence from a network meta-analysis. PLoS One. 2014;9:e99682.
64. Morsali M, Poorolajal J, Shahbazi F, Vahidinia A, Doosti-Irani A. Pharmaceutical therapies for the treatment of obesity: a network meta-analysis. Clin Ther. 2023;45:671–8.
65. Poorolajal J, Ghaleiha A, Darvishi N, Daryaei S, Panahi S. The prevalence of psychiatric distress and associated risk factors among college students using GHQ-28 questionnaire. Iran J Public Health. 2017;46:957–63.
66. Jahanshahi J, Hashemian F, Pazira S, Bakhshaei MH, Farahani F, Abasi R, et al. Effect of topical tranexamic acid on bleeding and quality of surgical filed during functional endoscopic sinus surgery in patients with chronic rhinosinusitis: a triple blinded randomized controlled trial. PLoS One. 2014;9:e104477.
67. Varkevisser CM, Pathmanathan I, Brownlee A. Designing and conducting health systems research projects: proposal development and fieldwork. Amsterdam: KIT Publishers; 1991.
68. Gilliland J, Clark AF, Kobrzynski M, Filler G. Convenience sampling of children presenting to hospital-based outpatient clinics to estimate childhood obesity levels in local surroundings. Am J Public Health. 2015;105:1332–5.
69. Salem W, Abdulrouf P, Thomas B, Elkassem W, Abushanab D, Rahman Khan H, et al. Epidemiology, clinical characteristics, and associated cost of acute poisoning: a retrospective study. J Pharm Policy Pract. 2024;17:2325513.
70. Ahmadpoor J, Mohammadi Y, Soltanian AR, Poorolajal J. Psychiatric disorders and associated risky behaviors among Iranian university students: results from the Iranian PDABs survey. J Public Health (Oxf). 2021;29:1197–204.
71. Zhong H, Zhou Y, Wang P, Jia Q, Wan Y, Xiong H. Influencing factors of bone mass abnormalities among postmenopausal women in Tibet. China BMC Public Health. 2023;23:2100.
72. Moeini B, Poorolajal J, Gharlipour Z. Prevalence of cigarette smoking and associated risk factors among adolescents in Hamadan City, West of Iran in 2010. J Res Health Sci. 2012;12:31–7.
73. Cheraghi P, Shahkolai FR, Poorolajal J, Hazavehi MM. Effect of educating mothers on injury prevention among children aged <5 years using the Health Belief Model: a randomized controlled trial. Public Health. 2014;128:825–30.
74. Ballini A, Gnoni A, De Vito D, Dipalma G, Cantore S, Gargiulo Isacco C, et al. Effect of probiotics on the occurrence of nutrition absorption capacities in healthy children: a randomized double-blinded placebo-controlled pilot study. Eur Rev Med Pharmacol Sci. 2019;23:8645–57.
75. Ho MS, Chow DH. Effects of kneeling posture on chest compression during cardiopulmonary resuscitation in males. J Clin Nurs. 2018;27:777–83.
76. Mazaheri S, Poorolajal J, Hosseinzadeh A, Fazlian MM. Effect of intravenous sodium valproate vs dexamethasone on acute migraine headache: a double-blind randomized clinical trial. PLoS One. 2015;10:e0120229.
77. Jahanshahi J, Pazira S, Farahani F, Hashemian F, Shokri N, Karkhanei B, et al. Effect of topical sucralfate vs clindamycin on Posttonsillectomy pain in children aged 6 to 12 years a triple-blind randomized clinical trial. JAMA Otolaryngol Head Neck Surg. 2014;140:698–703.
78. Azadbakht M, Razian A, Pooria A, Hadian B. Comparison of the effect of heparin, reteplase, and taurolock in the prevention of thrombosis in hemodialysis catheters. Health Sci Rep. 2024;7:e2057.
79. Khoshravesh S, Karimi-Shahanjarini A, Poorolajal J, Bashirian S, Barati M, Hamidi M, et al. Socio-cultural factors contributing to being an organ donor in Iranian employees. Community Health Equity Res Policy. 2022;42:171–9.
80. Kleinbaum DG, Sullivan KM, Barker ND. A pocket guide to epidemiology. New York: Springer; 2007.
81. Allo G, Sitarik AR, Redding A, Coleman CM, Cassidy-Bushrow AE, Gaba A, et al. Maternal COVID-19 exposure and placental characteristics. PLoS One. 2024;19:e0302682.
82. Mohammadian M, Omidi T, Shirmohammadi-Khorram N, Poorolajal J. Autism spectrum disorder and associated risk factors: a matched case-control study. Int J Epidemiol Res. 2019;6:14–9.

83. Smith AH, Kark JD, Cassel JC, Spears GF. Analysis of prospective epidemiologic studies by minimum distance case-control matching. Am J Epidemiol. 1977;105:567–74.
84. Pearce N. A short introduction to epidemiology. 2nd ed. Wellington: Center for Public Health Research; 2005.
85. Webb P, Bain C. Essential epidemiology: an introduction for students and health professionals. 2nd ed. New York: Cambridge University Press; 2011.
86. Wilson JA, O'Hara J, Fouweather T, Homer T, Stocken DD, Vale L, et al. Conservative management versus tonsillectomy in adults with recurrent acute tonsillitis in the UK (NATTINA): a multicentre, open-label, randomised controlled trial. Lancet. 2023;401:2051–9.
87. Hanrahan EJ, Madupu G. Epidemiology and biostatistics for the USMLE. New York: Appleton & Lange; 1994.
88. Elston RC, Johnson WD. Basic biostatistics for geneticists and epidemiologists: a practical approach. Chichester: John Wiley & Sons; 2008.
89. Hill AB. The environment and disease: association or causation? Proc R Soc Med. 1965;58:295–300.
90. Shadi Y, Heshmati B, Poorolajal J. Interaction between hepatitis B, hepatitis C, and smoking in the development of hepatocellular carcinoma: a systematic review and meta-analysis. J Public Health (Oxf). 2024;46:51–60.
91. Texas Children's Hospital. Toxic shock syndrome (TSS). 2024 [cited 16 Dec 2024].
92. Poorolajal J. Equivalence model: a new graphical model for causal inference. Epidemiol Health. 2020;42:e2020024.

MIX
Papier aus verantwortungsvollen Quellen
Paper from responsible sources
FSC® C105338

If you have any concerns about our products,
you can contact us on
ProductSafety@springernature.com

In case Publisher is established outside the EU,
the EU authorized representative is:
Springer Nature Customer Service Center GmbH
Europaplatz 3, 69115 Heidelberg, Germany

Printed by Libri Plureos GmbH
in Hamburg, Germany